CW01502302

The Beauty of Botanicals

By Tamara Warner

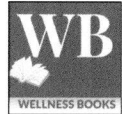

WELLNESS BOOKS

Copyright

The Beauty of Botanicals: Healing Plants for Wellness and Self-Care
Copyright© 2025 Tamara Warner. All rights reserved.

No part of this publication may be reproduced, stored in a retrieval system, or transmitted in any form or by any means — electronic, mechanical, photocopying, recording, or otherwise without the prior written permission of the copyright holder.

Published in the United Kingdom by Wellness Books
www.wellnessbooks.co.uk

This book was created with limited use of AI tools to support research and collation of information, with the text drafted, curated and approved by the author.

This book is for informational and educational purposes only. It is not intended to diagnose, treat, cure or prevent any disease. Always consult a qualified healthcare professional before using botanicals, essential oils, or making changes to your health routine, especially if you are pregnant, nursing, taking medication, or have a medical condition.

Cover design by Iain Hill of 1981D
ISBN: 978-1-0684581-3-2
First published 2025
Printed in the United Kingdom

The Beauty of Botanicals

Healing Plants for Wellness and Self-Care

By Tamara Warner

This book is dedicated to my fabulous mother, Monica Warner.

I'm so grateful for her support during the process of research and writing this book, her high standards of perfection, and also for her incredible knowledge and understanding of the wonderful world of horticulture and the fascinating potential of botanical healing.

To Mama, with love and light, thank you for everything.

Contents

Introduction

I'd describe myself as a passionate advocate of the extraordinary potential of herbal healing, in its many modalities. I specialise in aromatherapy and herbal apothecary, and through many years of research and development as a certified practitioner, became the creator of a range of therapeutic health and body products called Tamsorella's Botanicals.

Having been on an extensive journey of discovery into the world of herbology, I've experienced some of the most beautiful environments of the world: the Caribbean, English Cotswolds, the Mediterranean Islands, Greece and the Maldives, where I distilled my own essential oils and worked as wellness herbologist. Even so, I continue to be in awe when faced with the miraculous healing potential of some of the most common herbs, trees, roots, barks, resins, berries, fruits and flowers we see all around us, growing naturally in the wild, and in our gardens, conservatories and curated open spaces all over our world.

Over recent years, our social and cultural understanding of botanicals for wellness has experienced an exciting rebirth: as our daily existence becomes more complex, and our environments increasingly technological and time-pressured, the need for balance has become more paramount to our notions of well-being. As such, herbal practice at home is becoming more central to our everyday existence, as people search for healthy lifestyle choices and preventative, holistic medicinal solutions that can be grown, picked and prepared at home for family use.

I wrote this book to share the joys of my journey into the wonderful world of healing plants and to explain what I've learnt about herbology, in order to offer insight into these beautiful botanicals. It celebrates my experiences with healing herbs, plant oils and extracts, essential oils and hydrosols, offering information about botanicals and their usage in a way that makes it easy to understand and practice its teachings. The book contains personal observations, botanical profiles, recipes, applications and treatment suggestions; all of which I've practised myself, in my small studio in Greece.

My intention with this book is to demystify and explore the ways in which botanicals comfort, protect and nourish us, help us to heal and support our well-being. The process of learning simple botanical therapies and treatments has transformed the way I lead my life. As a result of these unique experiences, and in enormous respect of the natural plant world, as manifest in the very pages of this book, I invite you to delve deeper with me into the world of herbology.

The History of Herbal Medicine

What are herbs?

Herbs are plant materials humans have learnt to cultivate over thousands of years. Across the history of human development, we have eaten and used all possible plant parts as food and medicine – wild leaves, roots, shoots, flowers, seeds, nuts, fruits, berries, saps, gums resins, as well as bark.

We have developed in tandem with the natural world around us, our biological functions and processes having become attuned to the constituents within the plants. We have learnt when to use plants, how to use them, how much to use, and what their various features and properties are, including which plants will eventually kill us and which herbs will heal us best. Human biology has evolved in a symbiotic relationship with the plant kingdom since the very beginnings of our life on this planet.

A history of humans and herbalism

Human use of herbs and plants for healing has a rich history that spans all cultures and civilisations. The development of herbal medicine throughout the ages includes several milestones.

Before 3000 BCE – Prehistoric and Ancient

Pollen from medicinal plants found by archaeologists in the grave of a Neanderthal man dating back 60,000 years suggested that prehistoric humans may have used plants for medicinal purposes. It seems reasonable to assume that early humans would have learned about medicinal plants through trial and error, observation of animals and oral traditions shared from tribe to tribe.

Post-3000 BCE – the Sumerians

This era represents some of the earliest recorded uses of medicinal plants on clay tablets, where some 250 plants, including thyme and opium poppy, were documented.

C. 2800 BCE

The earliest Chinese medical text, called *Shen Nong Ben Cao Jing*, details the properties of 365 medicinal plants and is attributed to the mythical Emperor Shen Nong – the founder of Chinese medicine.

2000 BCE – the Ancient Egyptians

The Ancient Egyptians have left us with the *Ebers Papyrus* (circa 1550 BCE) – one of the oldest medical works – which lists more than 700 medicinal plants, including Aloe vera, garlic, cannabis and frankincense, which they famously used with bitumen and myrrh to mummify the dead bodies of their nobility; a testament to its properties of preservation.

1500 BCE

India

Ancient Indian texts such as the *Rigveda* and *Atharvaveda* mention the use of herbs underpinning Ayurveda, a comprehensive medical system that has contributed hugely to the foundations of holistic medical practice today. The texts list hundreds of medicinal plants, including ginger, turmeric and ashwagandha.

Ancient Greece

Known as the seat of Western civilisation from 500BC onwards, Greece gave us Aristotle and Hippocrates; the latter, known as the 'Father of Medicine', emphasised the use of herbs like willow bark for pain relief. Later, circa 500AD, Dioscorides, together with his apprentice Theophrastus, further documented the medicinal properties of plants, and promoted the path of wellness through nutritional and herbal remedies in their comprehensive literary and medicinal works.

The Middle Ages

During this period, written evidence of herbal medicine was primarily preserved and practised by monks and Islamic scholars. These male-dominated institutions played crucial roles in recording and developing herbal knowledge during the Middle Ages.

Herbal healing was practised in daily life mainly by women – wives, mothers, daughters and elders – as healers in the home. Of course, as women were generally excluded from recorded contributions to literature as well as academic institutions, these female healers of the Middle Ages had little opportunity to contribute to the science of medicine. Notwithstanding, they provided a fundamental role as herbalists, midwives, surgeons and traditional healers. As nuns in convents or simply within their own home, female healers notably used traditional botanical therapies and home remedies.

Hildegard of Bingen, a 12th-century Benedictine nun, was one of the most famous women in the herbal tradition at this time. She produced a comprehensive herbal medical text called *Causae et Curae*, in which she detailed her considerable herbal knowledge.

The 'Witch Craze': a horrific, historical era of slaughter between the 14th and 18th centuries across Europe, sustained partially by the Catholic church, and supported by the legal and medical professions. An estimated 80,000 women were put to death, most of whom were innocent young girls, older, unmarried women, healers, herbalists and midwives. This was primarily justified by a document entitled *Malleus Maleficarum*, conceived by two monks. Published circa 1484, it outlined an inescapable and complex system of the ways in which a witch could be identified, and was used to fuel a campaign of terror, burning, drowning and murder.

The Renaissance

Thankfully, the Renaissance brought a stable period of significant development and preservation in the field of herbal medicine. This era brought a revival of classical texts, the introduction of new plants through exploration, and contributions from visionary practitioners such as Paracelsus, Brunfels, Fuchs, and Culpeper.

These dedicated herbalists laid the foundations for modern herbal medicine, ensuring that knowledge of medicinal plants continued to evolve and spread.

Nicolas Culpeper

Most notable amongst these herbalists was Nicolas Culpeper (1616-1654), an English herbalist, physician and astrologer, whose literary and medical contributions include: *The English Physician* and *The Complete Herbal*, which were groundbreaking in making herbal knowledge accessible to the general public.

Culpeper translated medical texts from Latin into English, and provided detailed information on the uses of common plants and weeds to treat various ailments using delightful local names such as 'knitbone' (comfrey), 'self-heal' (*Prunella vulgaris*) and 'heartsease' (viola), to name but a few. He emphasised the importance of using locally available plants, and combined traditional herbal knowledge with astrological principles. His herbal manual is still in print today, providing a wonderful, historical snapshot of 17th-century English herbal medicine.

The decline of herbalism

Herbal medicine has deep roots in European history, serving as the mainstay of healthcare for centuries; however, with the onset of the Industrial Revolution in the late 18th century, things began to shift dramatically. Technological advancements spurred a new age of scientific inquiry, overtaking – and casting doubt on – traditional herbal practices.

A major blow to herbalism was the rise of modern chemistry and pharmacology. Scientists started isolating active compounds from plants, leading to the creation of more potent synthetic drugs. These lab-made medicines could be standardised, accurately dosed and mass-produced, making them seem more reliable than their herbal counterparts. The establishment of medical schools and professional institutions began to discredit herbalist traditions, calling them old-fashioned, and herbalists untrained when compared to formally educated doctors.

Meanwhile, early pharmaceutical companies, eager for profits, heavily promoted synthetic medicines that could be patented and sold en masse. For example, heroin – so called, it has been said, because of its ability to provide immediate pain relief – was deemed a hero in early 20th century; at that time, the medical establishment was unaware of the deadly, addictive nature of the chemical formulation.

4

Public health initiatives, especially in crowded urban areas, leaned heavily on vaccines and antibiotics to combat rapidly spreading diseases; in this context, herbal remedies, with their slower and more individualised approach, seemed inadequate.

Despite urbanisation distancing people from nature and traditional knowledge, herbal medicine did not vanish entirely; many continued to use herbal remedies alongside modern treatments. Yet, in the face of industrialisation, standardisation, growing populations and the pursuit of profits, the holistic nature of herbalism became at odds with the demands of modern life.

In essence, the decline of herbal medicine in Europe was a process influenced by scientific advancements, the rise of modern medicine, the influences of a developing pharmaceutical industry, and social changes brought about by industrialisation.

Modern-day usage of botanicals

Given the expansion of the last 100 years – in population and global commerce, and industry and its legalities, alongside rapid discovery, development and innovation within modern medical practice – it would be fair to say our relationship with the natural world of plants deteriorated. However, during the last fifteen to twenty years, there has been a noticeable awakening into wellness and self-care, and a search for alternative forms of medical and psychological healing to reduce the stress of our modern, technological working environments. This is coupled with a yearning for a deeper connection with our natural world.

This resurgence is part of a broader interest in natural and holistic approaches to health – demonstrating its enduring relevance in human healthcare.

Major benefits of herbal medicine

In an era when manufactured drugs dominate the healthcare industry, the merits of herbal medicine are often overlooked. However, there are compelling reasons to reconsider the role of herbal remedies in modern medicine, and to shift towards a more individual and home-oriented approach to wellness and health. There are a few reasons why this shift may have occurred.

Tried and tested over millennia

Herbal medicine has been in use for thousands of years. Modern medical practice and pharmaceuticals industries, on the other hand, have only been in existence for roughly 150 years. For example, Traditional Chinese Medicine (TCM), Ayurveda and Native American healing practices have been developed over millennia. Unlike many pharmaceuticals, which are relatively new and often tested for only a few years before being marketed, herbal medicines have stood the test of time, proving their efficacy across generations and cultures.

Preventative care

Herbal medicine focuses on a holistic approach to health, treating the individual as a whole rather than targeting isolated symptoms. This philosophy is rooted in the belief that physical, emotional and spiritual well-being are interconnected. By addressing the underlying causes of illness and promoting overall wellness, herbal medicine becomes preventative.

In addition, it excels in preventative health care by promoting long-term wellness. Many herbs possess adaptogenic properties, helping the body resist stressors and maintain balance; for example, herbs like ashwagandha, turmeric, Echinacea and ginseng are known to boost the immune system and to enhance resilience to stress. Incorporating these herbs into daily routines can fortify health and prevent illness, thereby reducing the need for pharmaceutical interventions.

Safety

One of the most significant advantages of herbal medicine is its typically lower incidence of side-effects when compared to pharmaceutical drugs; some synthetic medications can cause severe and debilitating side-effects.

Herbal remedies, being natural substances, are usually better tolerated by the body. For example, willow bark, lavender or peppermint used for pain relief are less likely to cause digestive and motility issues than the far more concentrated, prescribed pain-relieving drugs based on the original willow bark constituents. This makes herbal medicine a potentially safer option for long-term use.

Affordability

Using herbal medicine is often more affordable than pharmaceutical drugs, especially when you grow it yourself. Many medicinal herbs can be grown at home or purchased at a fraction of the cost.

Sustainability and environmental impact

The production of large-scale, manufactured pharmaceuticals causes pollution and depletes resources. Herbal medicine, when sourced sustainably, tends to have a much smaller environmental footprint. Growing medicinal plants can also promote biodiversity and support sustainable agricultural practices. In addition, herbal medicine aligns with the principles of eco-friendly living, as it encourages the use of natural resources in a responsible manner.

Empowerment through self-care

Using herbal medicine empowers individuals to take an active role in their health care; learning about medicinal plants fosters a deeper connection to nature and personal well-being. This empowerment can lead to better health outcomes, as individuals become more attuned to their bodies and proactive in maintaining their health. The ability to prepare and use herbal remedies also enhances self-sufficiency and reduces dependence on the healthcare system.

Synergy with the body's natural processes

Herbal remedies often work in synergy with the body's natural processes, supporting and enhancing the body's inherent ability to heal itself. This contrasts with many pharmaceuticals, which may interfere with, or override, natural bodily functions. For example, rather than blocking pain signals outright, certain herbs support the body's anti-inflammatory responses, promoting healing without significant disruption to normal physiological processes. This synergy can lead to more harmonious and sustainable health outcomes.

Addressing root causes of illness

Finally, herbal medicine often focuses on addressing the root causes of illness rather than merely alleviating symptoms. This comprehensive approach can lead to longer-lasting and more profound health improvements. For instance, rather than just lowering blood sugar levels, herbs used in TCM may aim to balance the entire endocrine system, thereby addressing the underlying imbalances that contribute to diabetes. This method contrasts with many pharmaceuticals, which focus on symptom control, potentially leaving the root cause unaddressed and leading to chronic dependency on medication.

In conclusion, the benefits of using herbal medicine in conjunction with, or as an alternative to, some over-the-counter pharmaceuticals are clear, and a lifestyle approach that integrates herbal remedies can often offer a balanced and enriched approach to health care and self-care.

All About Aromatherapy

While the use of aromatic plants is ancient, the development of aromatherapy as a distinct therapeutic discipline is rooted in more recent history. Aromatherapy, at its simplest, is the practice of using the concentrated, volatile oils of the natural plant for therapeutic benefit. 'Volatile' means that the oils will easily evaporate at room temperature – which is why we keep them stored away from heat and light, in dark-coloured bottles.

These essential oils are highly concentrated, aromatic compounds extracted from various parts of plants – flowers, leaves, stems, roots, bark or fruit rinds – typically through distillation or cold pressing. Due to their potency, they are never applied undiluted to the skin (except in the case of lavender and tea tree), and require careful handling and storage away from heat and light; generally in small, dark-coloured bottles with droppers through which the concentrated oils can be administered droplet by droplet – which can feel like a therapeutic act in itself.

Aromatherapy is a powerful plant-based therapy because it can offer instantaneous relief through the olfactory nerves, and is particularly useful for stress-related and emotional issues, due to this unique entry point into the body.

How does aromatherapy work?

It is fascinating that a simple inhalation of a synergetic essential oil blend can have such a profound effect on our minds and bodies. This is due to the clever connection between our sense of smell and the emotional control centre in our brain.

When you breathe in the aromatic molecules from an essential oil, they travel up your nose to a special area called the olfactory epithelium. Here, tiny sensory neurons grab onto these scent molecules, turning the aromas into electrical signals; what is really unique is that these signals then bypass the usual brain pathways and head straight to your olfactory bulb, which is like the brain's reception desk for smells.

From there, those signals get whisked away to the limbic system, a crucial part of your brain often called your 'emotional brain'. This system includes areas like the amygdala, which processes emotions and memory, explaining why a particular scent can instantly trigger a strong feeling or bring back a vivid memory. It also connects to the hypothalamus, which helps regulate everything from your heart rate to your stress response.

This direct line means essential oils can swiftly influence your mood, help you de-stress, kickstart your parasympathetic system of 'rest and digest', and even impact your body's overall balance – all by simply taking a breath. It is a beautiful example of how nature's chemistry can gently support our well-being.

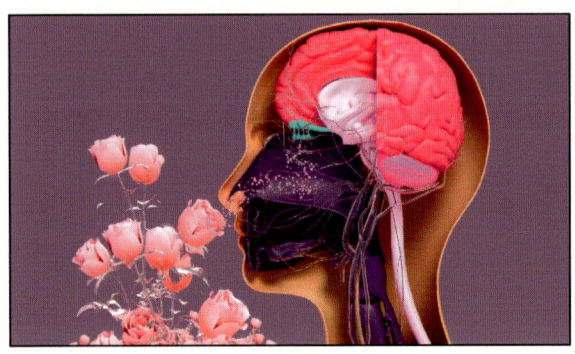

Due to this unique passage through the olfactory bulb and direct connection with the limbic system, the physiological effect of the inhalation can provide an immediate relief to feelings of stress, anxiety, grief or over-powering emotion. Certain oils, such as peppermint and rosemary, can also wake you up and instantly reduce that 'foggy brain' feeling. Other oils have an analgesic and anti-inflammatory action, so that a tiny drop applied topically can give instant pain relief and reduce swelling – excellent for insect stings and bites.

The origins of modern aromatherapy

The term 'aromatherapy' was coined in the early 20th century by French chemist René-Maurice Gattefossé, whose interest in essential oils stemmed from an incident in his laboratory circa 1910, when he reportedly burned his hand severely and plunged it into the nearest liquid – which happened to be lavender essential oil. He was fascinated to observe that the burn healed remarkably quickly, with minimal scarring. This personal experience spurred his scientific investigation into the properties of essential oils; particularly their antiseptic and healing capabilities. His research culminated in his seminal 1937 book, *Aromathérapie: Les Huiles Essentielles Hormones Végétales*, which laid the groundwork for modern practice.

Following Gattefossé's pioneering work, French physician Dr. Jean Valmet used essential oils to treat injured soldiers during the Second World War, documenting their therapeutic effects, particularly for wound healing and psychological support. At the same time, Austrian biochemist Marguerite Maury focused on the cosmetic and emotional applications of essential oils through massage, developing methods for their dilution and use in individualised treatments.

These three important figures, among others, were instrumental in shaping the clinical practice of aromatherapy as we understand it today, moving it from chemical curiosity to a distinct science called phytotherapy, or 'plant healing'.

How to use essential oils

There are several ways we can employ the power of plants. The primary methods of using essential oils in aromatherapy are:

Inhalation

This is the most direct route for influencing mood and the respiratory system. Inhalation can be passive, such as using a diffuser or simply opening a bottle and carefully sniffing; or active, such as a deep, steam inhalation, wonderful for bronchial or chest problems, or using an inhaler stick inside the nose.

Topical application

Applying essential oils to the skin allows for local effects such as reducing inflammation, pain relief, as well as soothing muscles, healing skin and potent systemic absorption, due to the tiny molecules which can penetrate the skin.

Essential oil molecules are incredibly small, allowing them to slip through the natural, protective layers of your skin; particularly the outermost stratum corneum, which acts like a brick wall. This layer is also rich in fats (lipids), and since essential oils are also lipophilic (meaning they mix well with fats), they can readily dissolve into, and pass through, this oily barrier.

*Essential oils must always be diluted in a carrier oil (such as sweet almond, jojoba, or coconut oil) before being applied to the skin, to prevent severe irritation and ensure safe absorption. They can be used for massage, baths, compresses or added to skincare products.

The vegetable-based carrier oil plays a vital role too; it dilutes the concentrated essential oil for safe application, helps it spread evenly, and most importantly, slows down the essential oil's evaporation, giving the molecules more time to penetrate the skin's surface and eventually enter your bloodstream, allowing their beneficial properties to work their magic throughout your body.

Internal consumption of essential oils is not recommended for the public and should only be undertaken under the strict supervision of a qualified medical practitioner or certified aromatherapist trained in this specific method, due to the potential for toxicity and damage to mucous membranes.

How is aromatherapy used?

Aromatherapy is primarily employed as a complementary therapy to support well-being and to address a range of common concerns. Its therapeutic potential is often explored in the following areas:

Stress reduction & mood enhancement

- Lavender
- Bergamot
- Chamomile
- Lemon
- Rosemary

- Lime
- Peppermint

Many essential oils – such as lavender, bergamot and chamomile – are widely used for their calming and anxiety-reducing properties. Others, like lemon, rosemary, lime and peppermint, are used to uplift mood and combat fatigue.

Inhalation is particularly effective for influencing emotional states via the limbic system.

Sleep support

- Lavender
- Frankincense
- Marjoram

Relaxing oils like lavender, frankincense and marjoram are frequently used to promote relaxation and improve sleep quality, often through diffusion in the bedroom or application to pulse points.

Respiratory support

- Eucalyptus
- Ravintsara
- Tea tree
- Peppermint

Certain essential oils, such as eucalyptus, ravintsara, tea tree and peppermint, are used via inhalation to help clear congestion and support respiratory function; often used in steam inhalations or chest rubs (diluted).

Skincare

- Tea tree
- Frankincense
- Calendula
- Chamomile

When properly diluted, some essential oils like tea tree (for blemishes), frankincense (for rejuvenation), calendula and chamomile (for soothing) are used to support skin health, due to their antiseptic, anti-inflammatory or regenerative properties.

Pain relief

- Lavender
- Eucalyptus
- Wintergreen
- Ginger
- Rosemary
- Peppermint
- Black Pepper

Topical application (in dilution) of oils like lavender, eucalyptus, wintergreen, ginger, rosemary, peppermint or black pepper may be used to help soothe topical and muscular aches and pains due to their anti-inflammatory and analgesic properties.

Aromatherapy offers an accessible and enjoyable pathway to enhance personal well-being. Rooted in early 20th-century scientific inquiry and evolving through continued practice and research, it provides a means to harness the concentrated, therapeutic power of plants. Through inhalation and topical application, essential oils can support emotional balance, promote relaxation and contribute to physical comfort, making aromatherapy a valuable and aromatic component of holistic self-care.

It is important to understand that aromatherapy is not a substitute for conventional medical treatment; however, it can serve as a valuable, complementary resource to support the body's natural healing processes.

Safety and professional guidance

While generally safe when used correctly, essential oils are potent substances. Key considerations include:

Dilution

Always dilute essential oils in a carrier oil before applying to the skin.

Quality

Use high-quality, pure essential oils from reputable suppliers.

Individual sensitivity

Perform a patch test before applying a new oil liberally to the skin.

Contraindications

Certain oils should be avoided in specific populations (e.g., pregnant women, young children, individuals with certain medical conditions).

For personalised advice, and to ensure safe and effective use, particularly for therapeutic purposes or if you have underlying health conditions, consulting a qualified and certified aromatherapist is highly recommended.

What is synergistic blending?

Imagine each essential oil as a uniquely therapeutic musical note, beautiful on its own – but when combined mindfully with others, they create a beautiful harmony, more soothing and musically intense than the sum of their individual parts.

This is the essence of synergy: when two or more essential oils are blended which have similar therapeutic constituents, the combined effect is made much more powerful, offering a deeper healing effect on the systems. As we navigate the slings and arrows of daily life, from managing stress and balancing hormones to nurturing emotional well-being and practising self-care, use of synergistic essential oil blends are a gentle yet powerful ally.

How does blending work?

Essential oils are made up of specific chemical constituents, each contributing to their therapeutic properties. The enhanced benefits of synergistic blending stems from the interaction of their volatile compounds.

Each essential oil contains a unique profile of molecules. These can be grouped together into monoterpenes, esters, aldehydes, and phenols, each with distinct physiological activities.

For instance, monoterpenes, often found in citrus and conifer oils, are celebrated for their uplifting and invigorating properties, with limonene in particular used for its antioxidant and cleansing effects. When blended, these compounds can work more strongly. Esters, which occur in oils such as lavender, wintergreen and chamomile, are blended for their calming and soothing influence on the nervous system; they promote relaxation, helping the body rest and restore.

Crafting beneficial aromatherapy blends involves careful consideration, moving beyond just a pleasing aroma to a deeper understanding of molecular contributions and effects. Aromatherapists carefully select oils whose principal constituents offer a broader spectrum of benefits when combined. For instance, a blend aimed at hormonal balance might combine oils rich in balancing esters with those containing sesquiterpenes, known for their grounding and anti-inflammatory properties, creating a more comprehensive effect. In the same way, to support emotional de-stressing, a blend might combine the uplifting nature of monoterpenes with the anxiety-reducing properties of aldehydes.

It is about creating a personal aromatic sanctuary, where the combined molecular effect of nature's most potent botanicals restore balance and foster a sense of peace and vitality.

Chemical constituents of essential oils

We now know that essential oils are composed of various chemical constituents, each contributing to their therapeutic properties. Below is a simple breakdown of the major chemical constituents found in essential oils, and their effects on the nervous system and other body systems.

1. Terpenes

Terpenes are hydrocarbons found in many essential oils, and are responsible for their distinct aromas. They have various therapeutic properties, including anti-inflammatory, antiseptic and analgesic effects.

Monoterpenes (e.g., Limonene, α-Pinene, β-Pinene)

- Limonene: Found in citrus oils, it has uplifting and mood-enhancing properties. It can reduce anxiety and improve focus.

- α-Pinene and β-Pinene: Found in pine and rosemary oils, these have anti-inflammatory and bronchodilator effects, helping to improve respiratory function.

Sesquiterpenes (e.g., β-Caryophyllene, Humulene)

- β-Caryophyllene: Found in clove and black pepper oils, it has anti-inflammatory and analgesic properties. It interacts with cannabinoid receptors, which can help reduce pain and anxiety.

- Humulene: Found in hops and coriander, it has anti-inflammatory and appetite-suppressant properties.

2. Phenols

Phenols are powerful antiseptics and stimulants. They have a warming effect and are known for their antibacterial and antiviral properties.

- Thymol: Found in thyme oil, it has strong antimicrobial properties and can help boost the immune system.

- Eugenol: Found in clove oil, it has analgesic and anti-inflammatory properties, often used for dental pain relief.

3. Esters

Esters are known for their calming and antispasmodic properties. They are often used to relieve stress and tension.

- Linalyl acetate: Found in lavender and bergamot oils, it has calming and anti-inflammatory properties, helping to reduce stress and improve sleep quality.

– Geranyl acetate: Found in citronella and rose oils, it has anti-inflammatory and sedative effects, promoting relaxation and emotional balance.

4. Alcohols

Alcohols in essential oils have antimicrobial and antiseptic properties. They are generally safe and non-irritating.

– Linalool: Found in lavender and coriander oils, it has calming and sedative properties, which can help reduce anxiety and improve sleep.

– Citronellol: Found in rose and geranium oils, it has antibacterial and anti-inflammatory properties, promoting skin health and reducing stress.

5. Aldehydes

Aldehydes have strong antimicrobial properties and can be calming or irritating, depending on their concentration.

– Citral: Found in lemon and lemongrass oils, it has strong antimicrobial properties and can uplift mood and improve mental clarity.

– Cinnamaldehyde: Found in cinnamon oil, it has antimicrobial and anti-inflammatory properties, often used for its warming and stimulating effects.

6. Ketones

Ketones are known for their mucolytic and regenerative properties. They can be helpful in respiratory and skin healing applications.

– Menthone: Found in peppermint oil, it has cooling and analgesic properties, providing relief from headaches and muscle pain.

– Thujone: Found in sage and thuja oils, it has antimicrobial properties but can be toxic in high concentrations, so it must be used with caution.

7. Oxides

Oxides have expectorant and decongestant properties, making them useful for respiratory conditions.

- 1,8-Cineole (eucalyptol): Found in eucalyptus and rosemary oils, it has strong expectorant properties, helping to clear respiratory passages and improve breathing.

Effects on the nervous system and other body systems

Nervous system

Calming and sedative effects

Esters (e.g., linalyl acetate, geranyl acetate) and alcohols (e.g., linalool) can reduce anxiety, promote relaxation and improve sleep quality.

Stimulant effects

Terpenes (e.g., limonene, α-pinene) and phenols (e.g., eugenol) can improve mood, enhance focus and provide a sense of alertness.

Respiratory system

Oxides (e.g., 1,8-Cineole) have decongestant and expectorant effects, helping clear nasal and bronchial passages to make breathing easier.

Immune system

Phenols (e.g., thymol) and aldehydes (e.g., chitral) have antimicrobial and antiviral properties: helping protect against infections by killing or inhibiting the growth of pathogens.

Musculoskeletal system

Terpenes (e.g., -caryophyllene) and ketones (e.g., menthone) have anti-inflammatory and analgesic effects, helping reduce inflammation and pain, providing relief from muscle and joint discomfort.

Skin

Alcohols (e.g., citronellol) and ketones (e.g., thujone) have regenerative and antimicrobial properties, promoting skin healing and protecting against infections.

What is the 'blending factor' in aromatherapy?

In aromatherapy, the 'blending factor', sometimes called the 'intensity factor', is a simple way to help you balance the aroma and strength of different essential oils when you are mixing them together.

Think of it like this:

- Some essential oils are very strong-smelling (e.g., peppermint, clove, lemon). Just one drop can dominate a blend.
- Other essential oils have a much lighter, more subtle scent (e.g., frankincense, sandalwood, rose). You might need many more drops of these for their aroma to come through.

The blending factor is a scale, usually from one to 10 (though some systems may vary), that rates an essential oil's aromatic intensity:

- Lower numbers (e.g., 1-3): Indicate very strong, potent oils. You will use fewer drops of these.
- Higher numbers (e.g., 7-10): Indicate lighter, more subtle oils. You will need more drops of these.

The goal is to use the blending factor to create a harmonious and pleasant smell, where no single oil overpowers the others, even if you want certain therapeutic effects to be dominant. So, if you are making a blend and want to use a strong oil like peppermint, and a lighter oil such as lavender, you would use fewer drops of peppermint relative to lavender oil, in order to achieve a balanced aroma.

The blending factor is a guideline to help you proportion your oils correctly, ensuring your blend smells good and has the intended effect, without being overwhelming or too faint. The following chart details the blending factors, and their uses, of the most common essential oils.

Essential Oil	Latin Name	Blending Intensity Factor (1-8, 1=most intense)	Commonly Blends With	Common Ailments Used For	Specific Ways of Application
Lavender	*Lavandula angustifolia*	7	Bergamot, chamomile, geranium, frankincense, lemon	Anxiety, insomnia, minor burns, cuts, insect bites, skin irritation, headaches, stress relief	Diffuse, topical (diluted on skin, pulse points, temples), bath
Peppermint	*Mentha piperita*	1	Lemon, rosemary, eucalyptus, tea tree, lavender	Headaches, nausea, indigestion, muscle aches, fatigue, respiratory congestion	Inhale (direct from bottle, diffuser), topical (diluted on temples, stomach, muscles), *avoid near face of young children*
Tea Tree	*Melaleuca alternifolia*	3	Lavender, lemon, eucalyptus, rosemary	Acne, fungal infections (nails, feet), minor cuts/scrapes, insect bites, cold sores, disinfectant	Topical (diluted on affected area), cleaning sprays
Lemon	*Citrus limon*	6	Lavender, peppermint, frankincense, eucalyptus	Uplifting mood, cleansing, digestive support, colds/flu, concentration	Diffuse, topical (diluted on chest/feet), cleaning solutions

Essential Oil	Latin Name	Blending Intensity Factor (1-8, 1=most intense)	Commonly Blends With	Common Ailments Used For	Specific Ways of Application
Frankincense	*Boswellia carterii*	5	Lavender, myrrh, sandalwood, bergamot, lemon	Skin rejuvenation, stress, anxiety, inflammation, respiratory issues, meditation	Diffuse, topical (diluted on skin, pulse points), inhale
Eucalyptus	*Eucalyptus globulus*	4	Peppermint, lemon, tea tree, rosemary	Respiratory congestion (colds, flu, cough), muscle aches, mental clarity	Diffuse, topical (diluted on chest/back), steam inhalation
Chamomile (Roman)	*Chamomile Nobile*	7	Lavender, bergamot, Clary sage, geranium	Anxiety, insomnia, skin irritation, digestive upset, muscle spasms	Diffuse, topical (diluted on skin, temples, stomach), bath
Rosemary	*Rosmarinus officinalis*	4	Lemon, peppermint, eucalyptus, lavender, tea tree	Mental fatigue, poor concentration, muscle aches, hair growth, respiratory issues	Diffuse, topical (diluted on temples, scalp, muscles), inhale

Essential Oil	Latin Name	Blending Intensity Factor (1-8, 1=most intense)	Commonly Blends With	Common Ailments Used For	Specific Ways of Application
Clary Sage	*Salvia sclarea*	6	Lavender, bergamot, geranium, sandalwood	Hormonal balance (menstrual discomfort, menopause), stress, insomnia, emotional balance	Diffuse, topical (diluted on abdomen, pulse points), bath
Bergamot	*Citrus bergamia*	7	Lavender, geranium, jasmine, frankincense, sandalwood	Anxiety, depression, stress, uplifting mood, skin conditions (acne, eczema – *photosensitive*)	Diffuse, topical (diluted, *avoid sun exposure after application*), bath
Geranium	*Pelargonium graveolens*	5	Lavender, bergamot, rose, Clary sage, frankincense	Hormonal balance, skin health (acne, aging, oily), emotional balance, insect repellent	Diffuse, topical (diluted on skin, pulse points), bath
Clove Bud	*Syzygium aromaticum*	1	Orange, cinnamon, frankincense, myrrh, peppermint	Toothache relief, pain relief, immune support, digestive issues (very strong)	Topical (highly diluted; tiny amount on toothache), diffuse (diluted with other oils for immune support)

Essential Oil	Latin Name	Blending Intensity Factor (1-8, 1=most intense)	Commonly Blends With	Common Ailments Used For	Specific Ways of Application
Cinnamon Bark	*Cinnamomum zeylanicum*	1	Orange, clove, frankincense, ylang ylang	Immune support, digestive issues, circulation, warming (very strong, highly irritating)	Diffuse (very small amounts, blended), topical (extremely diluted, *use with caution*)
Ginger	*Zingiber officinale*	4	Lemon, peppermint, Black pepper, bergamot	Nausea, motion sickness, digestive upset, muscle aches, inflammation	Inhale, topical (diluted on stomach, muscles)
Orange (Sweet)	*Citrus sinensis*	7	Lavender, lemon, frankincense, cinnamon, clove	Uplifting mood, anxiety, cleansing, digestive support, sleep	Diffuse, topical (diluted), cleaning solutions
Ylang ylang	*Cananga odorata*	4	Bergamot, geranium, sandalwood, jasmine, rose	Stress, anxiety, insomnia, blood pressure, aphrodisiac	Diffuse, topical (diluted on pulse points, neck), bath

Essential Oil	Latin Name	Blending Intensity Factor (1-8, 1=most intense)	Commonly Blends With	Common Ailments Used For	Specific Ways of Application
Sandalwood	*Santalum album*	8	Frankincense, myrrh, rose, ylang ylang, bergamot	Relaxation, meditation, skin health (dry, ageing), emotional grounding	Diffuse, topical (diluted on skin, pulse points), inhale
Juniper Berry	*Juniperus communis*	4	Cedarwood, cypress, lemon, grapefruit, rosemary	Detoxification, fluid retention, muscle aches, skin conditions	Diffuse, topical (diluted on stomach, muscles, affected skin)
Cypress	*Cupressus sempervirens*	5	Cedarwood, juniper berry, lemon, sandalwood, frankincense	Respiratory support, circulation, muscle spasms, emotional grounding	Diffuse, topical (diluted on chest, legs, muscles)
Myrrh	*Commiphora myrrha*	5	Frankincense, sandalwood, lavender, tea tree	Skin healing, oral health, meditation, immune support	Topical (diluted on skin, gums), diffuse

Essential Oil	Latin Name	Blending Intensity Factor (1-8, 1=most intense)	Commonly Blends With	Common Ailments Used For	Specific Ways of Application
Vetiver	*Vetiveria zizanioides*	2	Lavender, sandalwood, frankincense, patchouli	Grounding, anxiety, insomnia, ADHD support, skin regeneration	Diffuse, topical (diluted on feet, pulse points)
Patchouli	*Pogostemon cabli*	3	Sandalwood, cedarwood, vetiver, myrrh, lavender	Skin healing (acne, eczema, scars), emotional grounding, anxiety, insect repellent	Diffuse, topical (diluted on affected skin, pulse points)
Lemongrass	*Cymbopogon citratus*	2	Geranium, lavender, tea Tree, eucalyptus, cedarwood	Muscle aches, insect repellent, cleansing, mental clarity	Diffuse, topical (diluted on muscles, repellent spray)
Cedarwood	*Cedrus atlantica*	6	Sandalwood, frankincense, juniper berry, cypress	Grounding, relaxation, skin health, hair growth, respiratory issues	Diffuse, topical (diluted on feet, scalp, chest)

Essential Oil	Latin Name	Blending Intensity Factor (1-8, 1=most intense)	Commonly Blends With	Common Ailments Used For	Specific Ways of Application
Marjoram	*Origanum majorana*	3	Lavender, chamomile, bergamot, rosemary, eucalyptus	Muscle aches, tension, insomnia, respiratory congestion, stress	Diffuse, topical (diluted on muscles, chest, feet)
Thyme	*Thymus vulgaris*	2	Lemon, eucalyptus, rosemary, tea tree	Immune support, respiratory issues, cleansing (very strong)	Diffuse (sparingly, blended), topical (highly diluted on feet, chest)
Grapefruit	*Citrus paradisi*	6	Lemon, bergamot, peppermint, frankincense, geranium	Uplifting, cleansing, energising, fluid retention, appetite support	Diffuse, topical (diluted, *photosensitive*)
Oregano	*Origanum vulgare*	1	Lemon, thyme, tea tree, peppermint (use sparingly)	Powerful immune support, antiviral, antibacterial, antifungal (very strong, irritating)	Diffuse (very small amounts, blended), topical (highly diluted, *use with extreme caution, often on soles of feet*)

Essential Oil	Latin Name	Blending Intensity Factor (1-8, 1=most intense)	Commonly Blends With	Common Ailments Used For	Specific Ways of Application
Coriander Seed	*Coriandrum sativum*	4	Bergamot, frankincense, lemon, ginger, peppermint	Digestive support (bloating, gas), muscle aches, relaxation	Topical (diluted on stomach, muscles), inhale
Fennel (Sweet)	*Foeniculum vulgare*	3	Ginger, peppermint, lemon, basil	Digestive issues (gas, bloating, constipation), hormonal balance, appetite regulation	Topical (diluted on stomach), inhale

Plant Profiles & Recipes

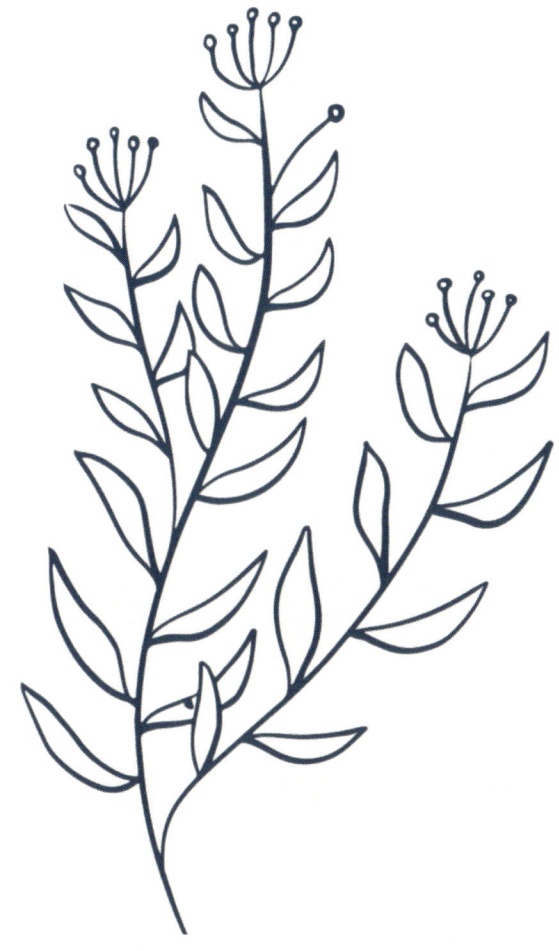

A Guide to Ingredients & Equipment

Here are some of my guidelines to follow to ensure the best results for your recipes.

Ingredients

If you don't have access to any of the specialist infused or pressed oils, such as infused chamomile, calendula, avocado, evening primrose, pomegranate or borage oil, then you can easily replace these with jojoba, sweet almond or coconut oil.

Try to source ethically sourced and organically produced, if at all possible.

Stockists

I source all the base ingredients and base oils I haven't produced myself, such as base face cream, cocoa butter, shea butter and Aloe gel, and essential oils which I don't or can't make myself, from Amphora Aromatics based in Bristol, UK. I've found them to be a reliable brand for an excellent range of organic, paraben-free, environmentally aware products.

You can find them at www.amphora-aromatics.com

Equipment

To make the recipes successfully, I recommend the following handy items:

- Chemistry set of 10 glass measuring beakers of various sizes, ranging from 5–500 ml.
  The small ones are important for creating the synergetic blends of essential oils, and the larger ones useful for measuring larger quantities and for mixing and blending your product.

- A Kilner jar – a brand of glass canning jar, known for its airtight seal created by a two-part lid, used for preserving and storing food.

- Measuring cylinders of 50–100 ml – ideal for pouring and measuring hydrosols and liquid vegetable oils.

- Glass rod stirrers are preferable for mixing bases and cold oils together.

- Silicon spatulas, useful for stirring heated and melted oils and butters.
- Glass Pasteur's pipettes are a must for precise droplet measurements for essential oils. I recommend buying a pack of ten, consisting of 5 x 5 ml and 5 x 10 ml pipettes.
- A set of cleaning brushes for small, glass chemistry cylinders is very useful.
- Glass bowls for bain marie – melting gently over simmering water in a pan – and for mixing and blending.
- Pack of silicone gloves to avoid getting essential oils on your fingers.
- Set of 20, 100 & 200-gram dark-glass cosmetics jars with lids, and lotion bottles with pumps.
- Electronic cosmetics weighing machine.

All of the equipment listed above can easily be bought online from Amazon or specialist stockists.

Measurements in the recipes

- Essential oils are measured drop by drop, and as a rule 20 drops = 1 ml. Some essential oils are more viscous and thicker than others; it's best practice to create your synergetic mixes in a small glass measuring cylinder, of 5, 10 or 15 ml, putting in drop-by-drop from the bottle, or using a pipette. Then you can swirl them around in the cylinder to mix before gently stirring with a glass rod.
- Hard butters, solid oils and infused oils are measured out in tablespoons, which I find easy to scoop out. Each tablespoon = approx. 15 grams of product on the weighing machine.

Where to make your products

If possible, product-making should be done in a workshop or utility room with sink, rather than in the kitchen, to avoid any contamination. I like to use a portable hot plate for the bain marie, in a simmering water pan. However, you can easily make the Elderberry Syrup and Echinacea Tincture in your kitchen, using kitchen pans.

Sanitisation

- Glassware is easily sanitised with rubbing alcohol available from any pharmacy.
- Using some form of preservative is very important when incorporating any substance containing water, such as hydrosol or Aloe gel, because water contains microbes. Using vitamin E alone as a preservative is not adequate. I recommend a natural preservative formulation such as preservative Eco /Geogard ECT (benzyl alcohol salicylic acid/glycerin sorbic acid). This is broad-spectrum preservative containing molecules found in nature.

  The rule of thumb here is to use as much as is necessary, in the smallest amount possible. In all the recipes in the book, 0.5 - 1% is enough. So, for example, if you're using 100 ml of water-based ingredient then you need to add 0.5 - 1 ml of preservative. However, if the product doesn't contain any water-based ingredients at all, then you don't need to add the preservative.

  Note: Most ready-made base cream and water-based products do contain preservatives, including those sold by Amphora Aromatics.

Safety when using essential oils

Essential oils are highly concentrated and you should wear silicon gloves when working with them, to avoid getting oil on your fingers – which could easily transfer to eyes, nose or mouth, where they could cause irritation.

Never put neat essential oil in your bath without mixing with a vegetable carrier oil first, as it will burn your skin – which can be a very unpleasant experience.

Essential oils that are labelled as photosensitive should never be applied when going out into the sun.

Labelling your recipes

As a general rule, all products should be carefully labelled including the date they were made.

Aloe vera

Aloe vera is a 'magical' plant valued worldwide for its ability to calm and sooth both nerves and including burns, wounds and skin irritations and is also a potent laxative due to the yellow latex found underneath the skin.

Latin name: *Aloe barbadensis miller*

Folk names: Burn plant, first aid plant, True aloe, Barbados aloe, Indian aloe, Lily of the Desert

Places of origin

The precise origin of Aloe vera has been the subject of much debate but it's widely believed to have originated in the Arabian Peninsula, and has naturalised in various tropical and subtropical regions around the world, including parts of Africa, India, the Mediterranean and the Americas. It thrives in arid and semi-arid climates.

Description

The Aloe vera plant has a remarkable resilience and striking form. At its core is a rosette of thick, fleshy leaves that spiral outwards like tentacles from a central point; their surface a matte, waxy green that can range from a deep jade to lime green, to minty-grey, often speckled or striped with lighter spots when young.

These deeply succulent leaves, plump, with a cooling, translucent gel, have a smooth, tough exterior and are lined with soft, protective teeth along their edges.

As the plant matures, a tall, elegant stalk can emerge, bearing a cluster of tubular flowers in shades of yellow and orange, creating a vibrant, torch-like flourish against the plant's stoic, green base.

Medicinal uses

Aloe vera contains vitamins A, C and E, which act as antioxidants and support the production of collagen within the skin. It's renowned for its soothing and healing properties, which is primarily attributed to the gel

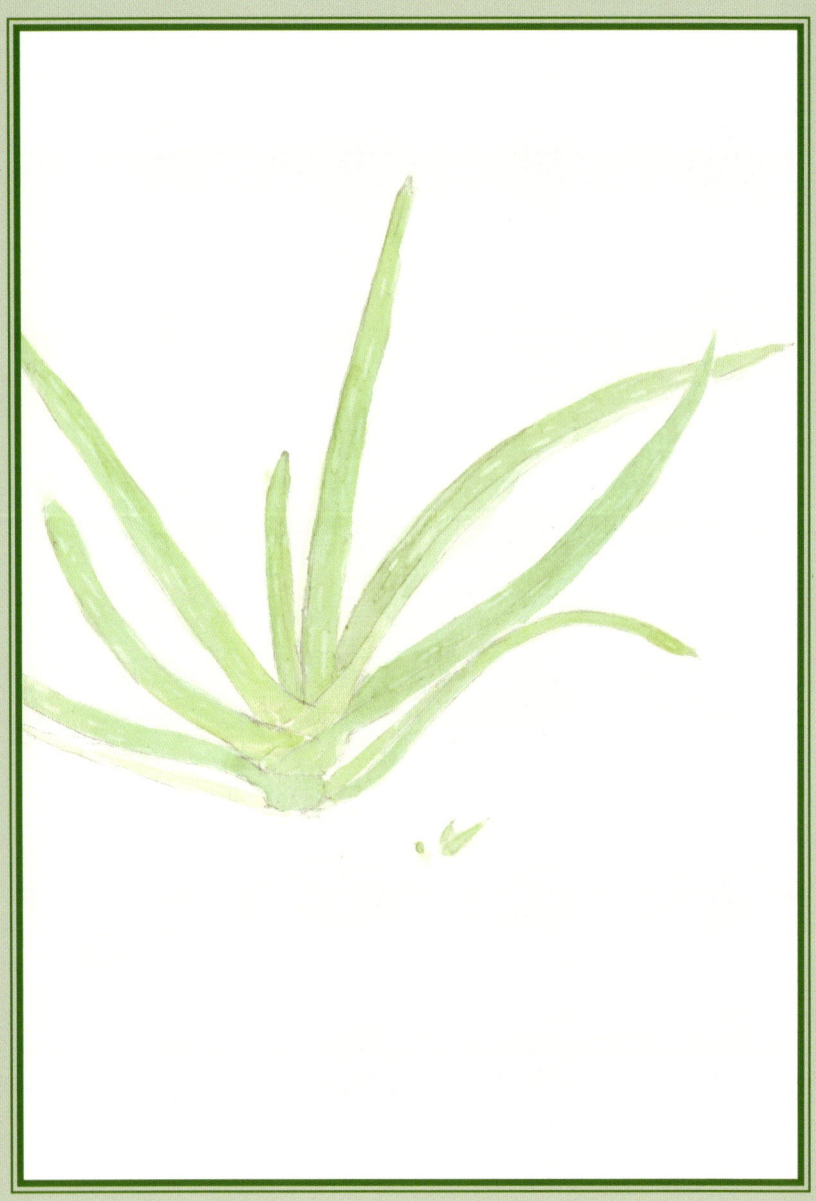

Aloe barbadensis miller

found within its leaves. Traditional and current usage has remained the same, including:

- ✓ Skin healing: Its gel is widely applied topically to soothe and promote the healing of burns (including sunburn), minor cuts, scrapes, insect bites and skin irritations. It helps to reduce inflammation, pain and the risk of infection.
- ✓ Moisturising: The gel is an excellent natural moisturiser for the skin, helping to hydrate and improve elasticity.
- ✓ Anti-inflammatory: Both topical and internal (with caution) use may offer anti-inflammatory benefits.
- ✓ Wound healing: Aloe vera can help to speed up the healing process of wounds by promoting cell regeneration.

Spiritual benefits

Aloe vera carries a gentle, yet potent, energy, often associated with:

- – Soothing and calming: Its energy is deeply soothing, helping to alleviate irritation and promote a sense of peace and well-being, mirroring its physical effects on inflamed tissues.
- – Healing and regeneration: Aloe embodies the energy of healing and renewal, supporting the body's natural ability to repair and regenerate.
- – Protection: Some traditions associate Aloe vera with protective energies, warding off negative influences and promoting a healthy energetic field.
- – Resilience: Its ability to thrive in harsh environments reflects an energy of resilience and adaptability.

Associated chakras

Solar Plexus chakra: This chakra is the centre of personal power, will and digestion – so, with its soothing effect on the digestive system and ability to promote healing and resilience, Aloe vera resonates with the balanced energy of this chakra, fostering inner strength and vitality.

Heart chakra: Its calming properties can also gently influence the Heart chakra, promoting emotional soothing and care.

Tamara's Tales: Aloe vera

I first encountered Aloe vera in Jamaica as a young girl of seven or eight. We were living in Trinidad and holidaying with family in Jamaica. I remember seeing tourists in some pain, having been burnt magenta by the hot sun. The Jamaican hotel owners were cutting and applying fresh strips of shining Aloe vera gel from the tall, fleshy plants outside. I was told the aloes were used to stop the burn going deeper, and to heal and protect the inflamed skin. 'A magical plant', I thought then – and still do now!

I grew these plants with great success in Greece, but the best specimens I've personally seen were in the Canary Islands in Lanzarote's ornamental cactus gardens: five feet tall with magnificent yellow, flowering spikes.

Recipe: Aloe vera skin soother

My recipe for Aloe vera is a soft, skin-soothing gel, which I created in Greece for clients and guests as a gentle after-sun skin soother and calming face mask.

What you'll need:

- 30 ml fresh Aloe vera gel
- 30 ml rose hydrosol (floral water)
- 3 drops lavender essential oil
- 1 drop peppermint essential oil
- 2 drops rose geranium essential oil
- 1 drop vitamin E oil
- 1 tablespoon chamomile- or calendula-infused oil if available; otherwise, replace with avocado or jojoba oil

Method:

1. Place all ingredients in a glass bowl or measuring beaker.
2. Blend together using a small, cosmetics hand-held stick blender until opaque and combined into a thick, creamy, gelled consistency.
3. Scrape into a clear, 100 ml glass cosmetics jar.
4. Place in the fridge.

Storage & expiry

Use within three days (due to the water content in the hydrosol and Aloe gel).

Borage (starflower oil)

Borage is known to be uplifting, while its oils have the potential to relieve symptoms of menopause, balance hormones and reduce inflammation.

Latin name: *Borago officinalis*

Folk names: Starflower, bee bush, bee bread, cool tankard, burrage

Places of origin

Native to the Mediterranean region, but naturalised in many parts of the world.

Description

Borago officinalis, known as 'borage', or 'starflower', grows freely across southern Europe and the Mediterranean region, and has been cultivated widely as a culinary and medicinal herb. It's unassuming, yet startling beautiful, producing abundant flowers.

Often described as a 'robust annual herb', it grows about half a metre in height with relatively large, hairy leaves and purple stems topped with delightfully blue, star-shaped flowers – larger or smaller, depending on the variety. The flowering tops are called *'Boraginis flos'* and yield its powerful seed oil, known commercially as Starflower oil.

Commonly seen as a hedgerow or wild border plant in the UK, up to two grams of the dried flower tops can be taken in a tea no more than three times a day for short-term use, acting as a mild sedative and antidepressant, and also capable of reducing high temperatures when taken hot, called a 'diaphoretic effect'.

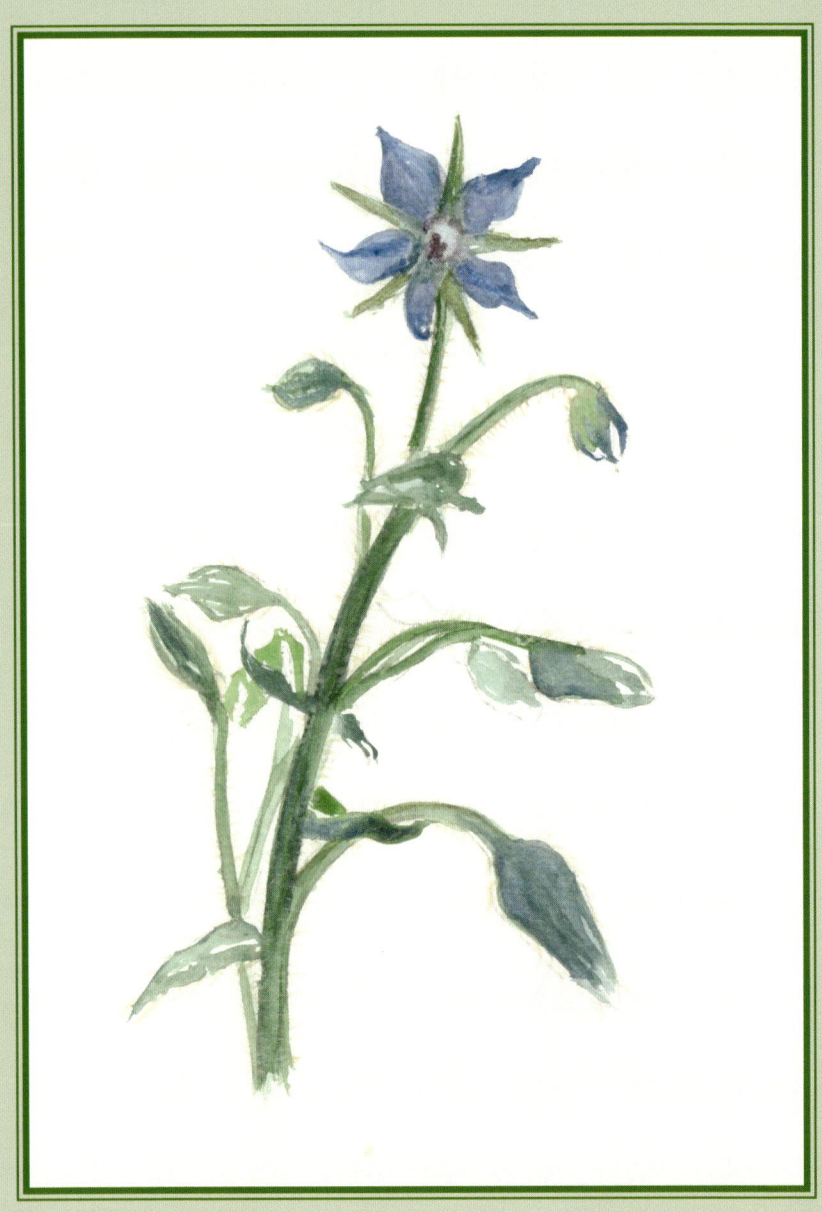

Borago officinalis

The Romans called Borage '*Euphrosynum*' – 'the plant that cheers'; and in Welsh, it translates as 'herb of gladness'.

Medicinal uses

The flower seeds of this plant are pressed into a wonderful oil, rich in essential fatty acids. Containing over 21% GLA, an omega 6 fatty acid called gamma-linolenic acid, it has a wealth of health benefits including:

✓ Reducing inflammation, boosting the immune system and supporting hormonal balance).

✓ Help regulating the prostaglandins that influence inflammation and mood, often used to alleviate symptoms of PMS and menopause.

✓ Traditionally used to support adrenal health and as a diaphoretic (promoting sweating) to help with fevers.

Contraindications

Studies suggest that dried borage should not be taken long-term and avoided during pregnancy.

Spiritual benefits

Uplifting, joyful, courage-enhancing, refreshing.

Associated with resilience, peace of mind, and the ability to lift a heavy heart.

Associated chakras

Heart chakra: Traditionally seen as a 'herb of gladdening the heart', promoting courage and emotional well-being.

Tamara's Tales: Starflower oil

Borage was one of the early annual wild spring herbs to adorn the perimeters of our olive grove and herbal terraces while I was living in Greece, producing masses of gently nodding buds atop delicate, swan-necked stems, atop a central branching shoot.

During my work as a herbologist there, I explored the capacity of borage oil in supporting menopausal symptoms of anxiety when combined with evening primrose oil and other phytoestrogenic essential oils (i.e. plants whose chemical constituents are similar to oestrogen), such as rose geranium and clary sage, alongside calming and relaxing essential oils such as lavender, ylang ylang and neroli.

I created a simple massage blend and roller ball preparation for myself and my clients aiming to encourage feelings of calm and relaxation, and help to reduce feelings of tension and anxiety. We had improved sleep as a consequence of using it.

Recipe: Anxiety relieving massage oil/roller ball blend (for menopause)

Roll on this anxiety-busting blend and breathe in deeply whenever you feel the need for a moment of calm.

What you'll need:

- 2 tablespoons borage seed oil
- 2 tablespoons evening primrose seed oil
- 5 drops clary sage essential oil
- 5 drops rose geranium essential oil
- 5 drops lavender essential oil
- 5 drops neroli essential oil
- 3 drops ylang ylang
- 2 tablespoons jojoba oil

Method:

1. Mix all oils well together and then add the synergetic essential oil mix.
2. Stir well and decant into a dark, glass bottle.
3. Carefully pipette the oil blend into clean roller ball dispensers for daily use; or simply use for massage on abdomen and lower back when needed.

Storage & expiry

Store in a cool, dry place and use within one year.

Calendula

Flowering year round, this joyous orange plant is renowned for its antiseptic qualities, which make it useful for wound-healing, and is also used to support digestion.

Latin name: *Calendula officinalis*

Folk names: Pot marigold, Garden marigold, English marigold, ruddles, gold-bloom

Places of origin

Native to Southern Europe, Western Asia and the Mediterranean.

Description

'Flower of the Sun', the beautiful, bright-orange colour of calendula brings joy and summer sweetness to everyone's garden. In fact, the name 'calendula' comes from the Latin word *'calendae'*, which means 'the first day of the month'. This name was given to the flower because it was known for its long blooming season.

In mild climates, calendula can bloom almost year-round, appearing to be in flower at the start of most months, like a natural calendar. The name is a diminutive, so it can be interpreted as 'little calendar' or 'little clock'.

Medicinal uses

- ✓ Highly valued for its remarkable wound-healing, anti-inflammatory and antiseptic properties; thus, widely used topically for cuts, scrapes, burns, rashes, insect bites and various skin irritations.
- ✓ Internally, it acts as a lymphatic cleanser and can be used to support digestive health and immune function.

Spiritual benefits

Warming, bright, protective, uplifting, healing.

Associated with comfort, vitality and bringing joy.

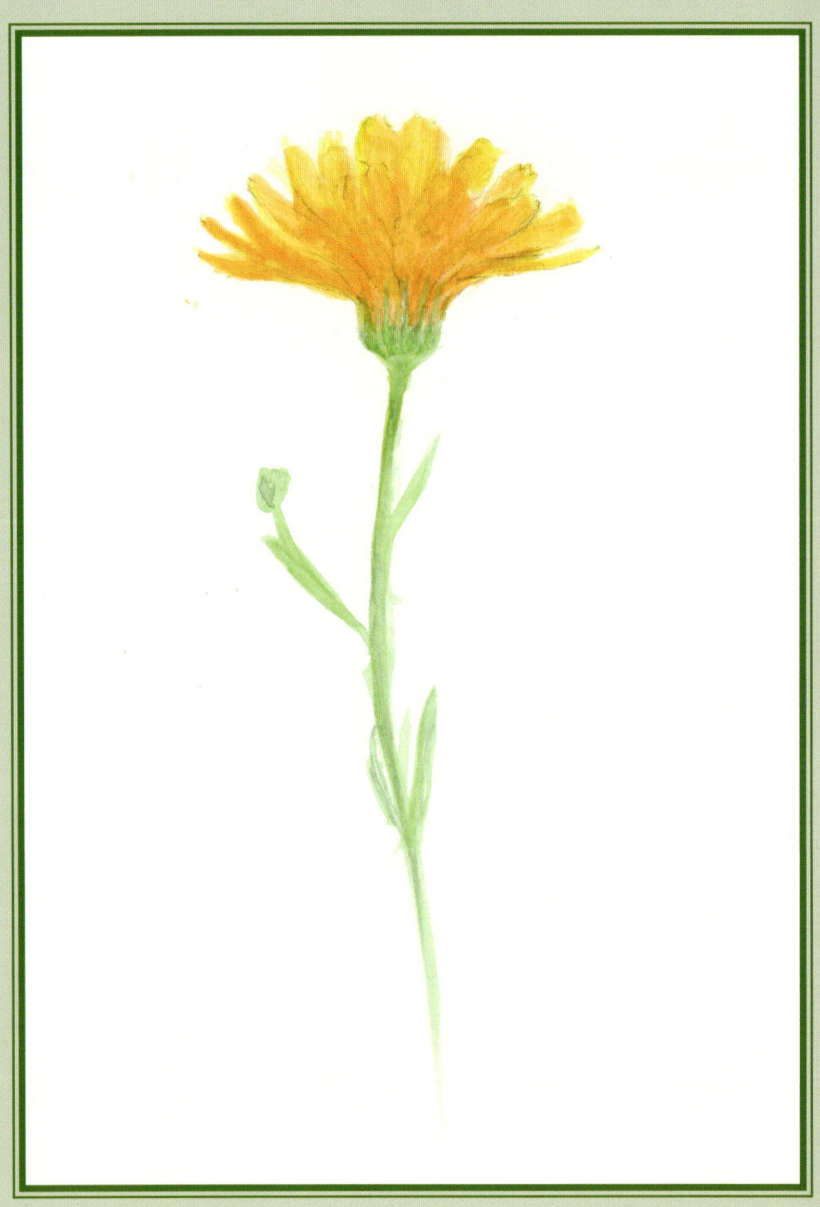

Calendula officinalis

Associated chakras

Solar Plexus chakra: Its warming and strengthening properties support digestion and personal power.

Sacral chakra: For its role in healing and promoting emotional flow.

Tamara's Tales: Calendula

In springtime in Greece, the mountainsides where I lived were covered with *Calendula avensus* – wild calendula – and I'd scramble excitedly over the rocky terrain, gathering the flowering tops in wicker baskets.

I dried out the residual moisture from the beautiful flowers for a couple of days on tabletops, and then stuffed them into mason jars, covering them with olive oil making sure all flower parts were fully immersed. The jars would sit outside in the full sunshine for a month or so, until the oil absorbed the deep-orange hue and the medicinal constituents from the flowers.

Finally, my calendula-infused oil was ready to strain off using a muslin bag, and poured carefully into jars and stored in my apothecary for creams, balms, lotion bars and beautiful bath oil treats.

Recipe: Calendula & chamomile skin-soothing cream

This luxurious cream is perfect for sore or irritated skin.

What you'll need:
- 2 tablespoons of Calendula infused oil
- 1 tablespoon of chamomile infused oil
- 1 teaspoon of St John's wort balsam*
- 1 ml (20 drops) of lavender essential oil
- 5 drops chamomile essential oil
- 4 tablespoons of organic base cream
- 50 ml of rose or lavender hydrosol
- 5 drops benzoic acid naturally derived preservative
- 4 drops vitamin E oil

* If you're taking any medication for example contraceptives or blood thinners then leave out the St John's wort, as it has a tendency to flush out other medications from the body. Replace with avocado oil.

Method:

1. In a medium sized glass bowl measure out the base cream and infused oils and gently mix together.
2. Next, add the lavender essential oil and stir well.
3. Add the vitamin E oil and the benzoic acid.
4. Drizzle the hydrosol into the mixture and whip till light and fluffy with either a small hand blender or an electric whisk.
5. Pipe or scrape your cream into two or three 100 ml dark-glass face cream jars.

Storage & expiry

Store in a cool, dry spot. Use within six months.

Clary sage

Clary sage is known for its powerful effects on the endocrine system and reputation for supporting menstrual as well as menopausal symptoms.

Latin name: *Salvia sclarea*

Folk names: Clear eye, see bright, eyebright, clary wort, oculus Christi

Places of origin

Native to the Mediterranean Basin and parts of Central Asia.

Description

Clary sage is a gorgeous, large-leaved biannual with beautiful creamy-white lilac and pink floral spikes. Its scent is strong and not to everyone's palette... however, I love it!

In herbal lore, clary sage is celebrated as 'the woman's oil', due to the fact it contains natural esters that are powerfully antispasmodic and appear to have an adaptogenic effect on the endocrine system – making it particularly effective for menstrual discomfort and mood regulation.

Medicinal uses

✓ Traditionally used for its calming and uplifting effects, particularly for stress, anxiety and insomnia.

✓ Known for antispasmodic properties, making it useful for muscle cramps and menstrual discomfort.

✓ In herbal medicine, often used as a tonic for the female reproductive system and to support hormonal balance.

Spiritual benefits

Euphoric, relaxing, visionary, cleansing, clarifying.

Associated with spiritual insight, creativity and dream work.

Associated chakras

Sacral chakra: Primarily associated with this chakra due to its connection with creativity, emotions and the reproductive system.

Third Eye chakra: Linked to this chakra for its ability to enhance intuition and spiritual vision.

Tamara's Tales: Clary sage

Clary sage grew in profusion in my herbal garden in Greece. The funny thing about the plant is that it'd never grow where I wanted it to; it preferred to spread out from my carefully delineated beds and grow everywhere else: in the gravelled walkways, and crevasses in the huge stony boulders, in particular.

I grew Clary sage for its beauty as well as its medicinal value, to distil its essential oil; I wanted to try it in a whipped balm to support the strong menopausal symptoms I was experiencing at that time.

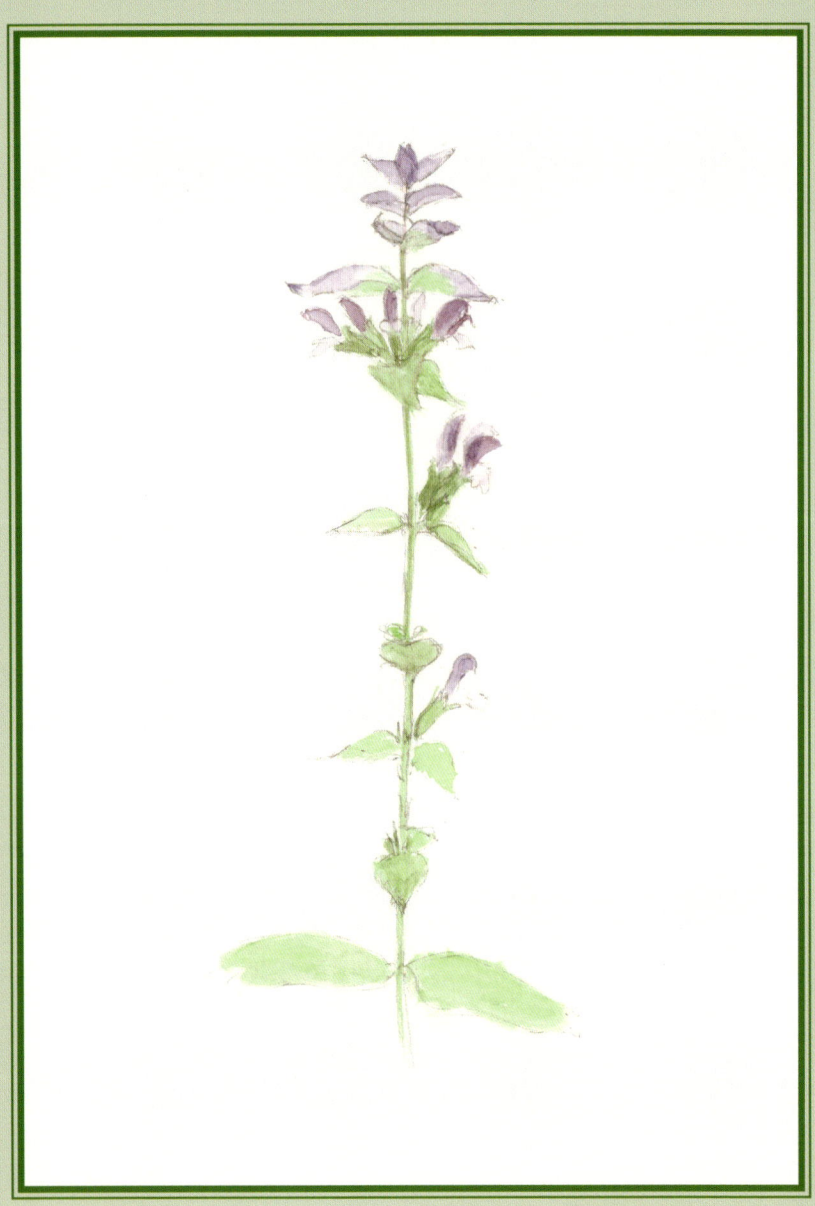

Salvia sclarea

It was an excellent addition to my herbal apothecary and due to its independent nature, I called the balm Artemis – after the fiery Greek goddess of the forest who turned Actaeon into a stag which was devoured by his obedient hounds, thinking he was their prey instead of their master. Artemis caused Actaeon's death because he'd intruded unwittingly upon her private solitude with her nymphs while bathing leisurely in a woodland glade: a powerful reminder never to disturb a woman in her bath!

Recipe: Artemis balm

My whipped balm is perfect for soothing hormonal issues and can be used as a body cream or a sumptuous massage balm.

What you'll need:

- 75–100 ml rose hydrosol
- 2 ml Clary sage essential oil
- 1 ml lemon verbena essential oil
- 2 ml lavender essential oil
- 1 ml rose geranium essential oil
- 1 tablespoon cocoa butter
- 2 tablespoons shea butter
- 1 tablespoon organic beeswax
- 1 tablespoon evening primrose oil
- 1 tablespoon borage oil
- 5 drops benzoic acid preservative*
- A few drops vitamin E

Note: The benzoic acid and vitamin E are very important in order to preserve the balm, as we've added hydrosol (flower water) to the mixture, which contains microbes.

Usually, if you buy a pre-prepared hydrosol, it will already contain a preservative; however, I'd advise adding 1% natural preservative for safety.

Method:

1. Gently melt together the beeswax and cocoa butter and the oils together in a bain marie.

2. Add the shea butter last, when ingredients have melted together.

3. Take off the heat, allowing to cool slightly before adding the synergetic mix of essential oils, and stir well whilst continuing to cool.

4. Add the benzoic acid and the vitamin E drops.

5. To create the creamy, whipped balm, carefully drizzle in the rose hydrosol whilst whipping with a small, handheld electric whisk or blender until the mixture is creamy, light and fluffy. You may not need to use all the rose hydrosol.

6. Carefully scrape the mixture into a piping bag and pipe into couple of 109 ml dark face cream glass jars, or simply scrape straight into the jars and pop the lids on.

7. Allow to cool.

8. Use with joy as a body cream, or massage balm on abdomen and lower back.

Storage & expiry

Keep in cool, dry area. Use within six months.

Echinacea (Purple coneflower)

While the entire Echinacea plant has beneficial properties, its root is considered the most potent part by many herbalists, being rich in active compounds known as alkylamides – believed to be responsible for the plant's renowned immune-boosting benefits.

Latin name: *Echinacea purpurea*

Folk names: Purple coneflower, Eastern Purple coneflower

Places of origin

Native to the eastern and central parts of North America, thriving in open environments like prairies and woodlands.

Description

The flowers of the Echinacea are striking and intriguingly structured: the huge, central cone is iridescent and multicoloured in a coppery-brown, deep orange and purplish-bronze with large, pink and purple petals draping down in an elegant reflex.

The cones resemble a small, spiky hedgehog – and, in fact, the name 'Echinacea' comes from the Greek word for hedgehog, *'echinos'*.

Although both its leaves and flowers are used, preparations focusing on the root – particularly from mature plants – are often considered superior in supporting the immune system.

Medicinal uses

✓ Immune-boosting

Scientific studies have shown Echinacea to be effective in fighting off upper respiratory infections like the common cold. Taking it when symptoms first appear can help shorten duration of illness and make the symptoms less severe. Thought to work by boosting activity of key immune cells and helping the body fight off germs more effectively.

✓ Contains compounds that can help reduce inflammation in the body, and may also have a direct effect against certain bacteria and viruses. A great ally for overall wellness, especially during cold and flu season.

Usage methods:

The most effective methods for preparing Echinacea root to capture these compounds include:

– Tinctures: Soaking the chopped root in alcohol and water is a highly effective way to extract the active components.

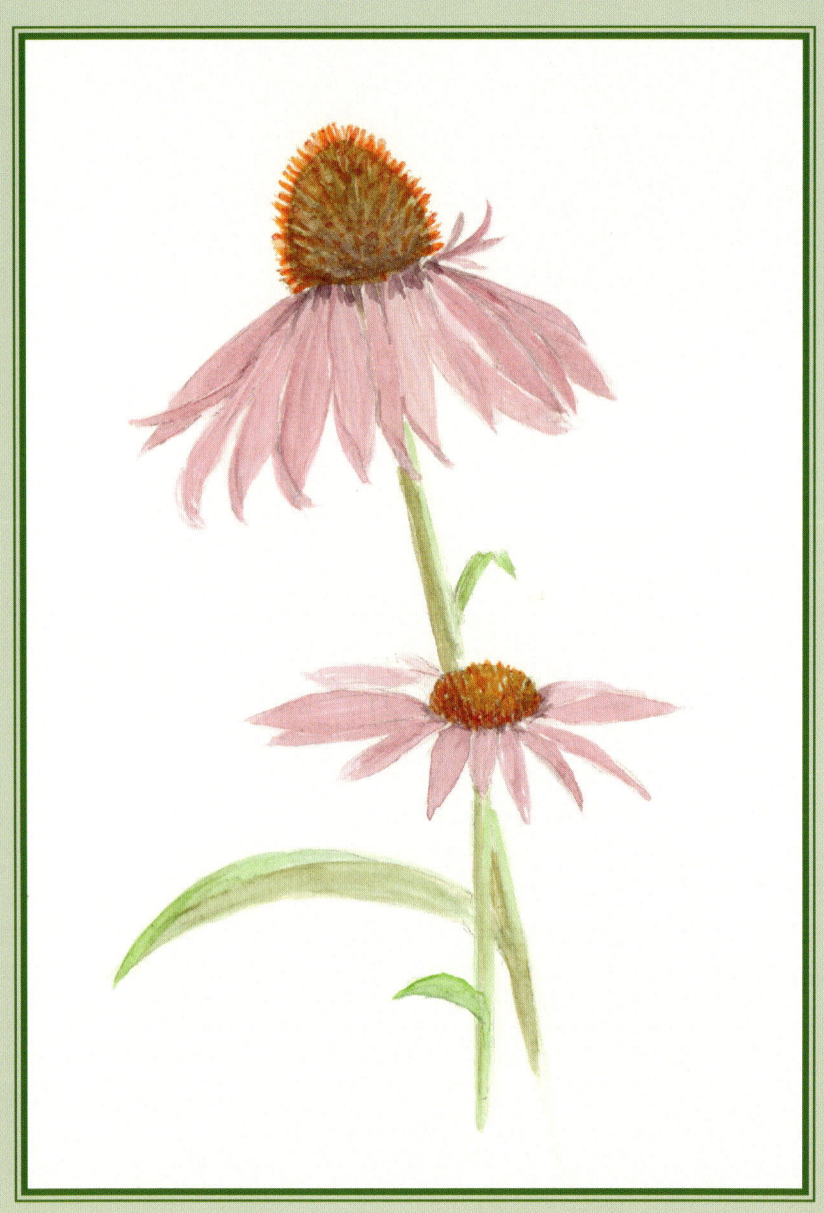

Echinacea purpurea

- Decoctions: Simmering the dried root in water can also be used to release its medicinal properties (note: some compounds may be affected by the heat).
- Capsules and tablets: Many commercial supplements contain standardised root extracts to ensure a consistent dose of key active ingredients.

Spiritual benefits

Energetically, Echinacea is associated with strengthening boundaries, promoting resilience and inner strength, and activating the body's natural defences.

Associated chakras

Root chakra: Associated with this chakra for its connection to physical strength and grounding.

Solar Plexus chakra: For its ability to boost vitality and self-efficacy.

Throat chakra: Due to its traditional use for throat ailments.

Tamara's Tales: Echinacea

I first bought my Echinacea seeds from a wonderful shop called Jekka's herb farm in Bristol years ago, for my 'great Greek escape' – an extensive farm run by an outstanding herb grower called Jekka.

I planted the seeds after Christmas, as I'd read they need to be scarified (frozen) to germinate. By the time I returned to Greece's Southern Peloponnese region after the spring school term, having left them in the capable hands of our handy man, the plants were well underway thanks to the help of another Albanian worker friend, who was an expert stone mason and had built two enormous, three-foot raised beds for them.

The plants eventually grew into magnificent specimens, underplanted with peppermint and interspersed with ginger.

A magnet for pollinators, my Echinacea grew so strongly that after two years, it had populated the entire raised bed and produced magnificent roots for herbal preparation.

Recipe: Echinacea immunity tincture

My Echinacea recipe is a powerful tincture to protect against viral illness and to support the body's recovery more quickly. Take a teaspoonful twice daily when you feel as if a cold, cough or viral infection is coming on.

What you'll need:

- 100 grams of dried Echinacea root
- 50 grams of wilted wild thyme
- 50 grams of dried oregano
- 100 grams of chopped fresh ginger root
- 50 grams of dried berries of sea buckthorn
- 2 litres strong vodka
- 10 large bay leaves

Method:

1. Place the prepared ingredients into a three-litre Kilner jar and cover with the strong vodka.
2. Leave in a cool dark place for three months, shaking the mixture up a little from time to time, to ensure all plant parts are equally distributed in the maceration.
3. When the maceration time is up, strain into a cheesecloth and carefully decant into sanitised, 100 ml glass bottles.
4. Label.

Storage & expiry

Keep cool and dry. Use within two years.

Testimonial

'The Echinacea Tincture works as a teaspoon of good, natural-tasting preventative – magic at the first signs of a cold, and contributes to reducing any development of the unpleasant symptoms.'

Catherine Chamier

Elder tree

The Elder tree produces a powerfully medicinal punch from both its flowers and berries. Its benefits have been used for centuries in tea infusions and compresses, and include immune-boosting properties and relief from cold symptoms.

Latin name: *Sambucus nigra*

Folk names: Elderberry, European elder, Black elder, Bore tree, Bour tree, Hylder, Eller, Holunder

Places of origin

Native to Europe, North Africa, and parts of Asia. It thrives in hedgerows, woodlands, and disturbed ground throughout these regions, including the UK.

Description

When in bloom, typically from late May to early July in the UK, pink-flowered elders present a spectacular contrast to surrounding trees. The umbel-shaped flowerheads are composed of numerous tiny blossoms, each tinged with shades ranging from a soft blush pink to deep, vibrant rose, which pop against the rich backdrop of its dark foliage.

Its delicate petals release a distinctly sweet, heady and slightly musky fragrance which fills the air, attracting a buzzing array of pollinators.

The Elder tree has been steeped in folklore and spiritual significance for centuries, often seen as a powerful threshold guardian and a connector between worlds – both beloved by the Celts and famed as part of Hippocrates medicine chest.

Medicinal uses

Elderflower:

- ✓ Traditionally used for colds, flu and respiratory issues due to its diaphoretic (promoting sweating) and anti-inflammatory properties.

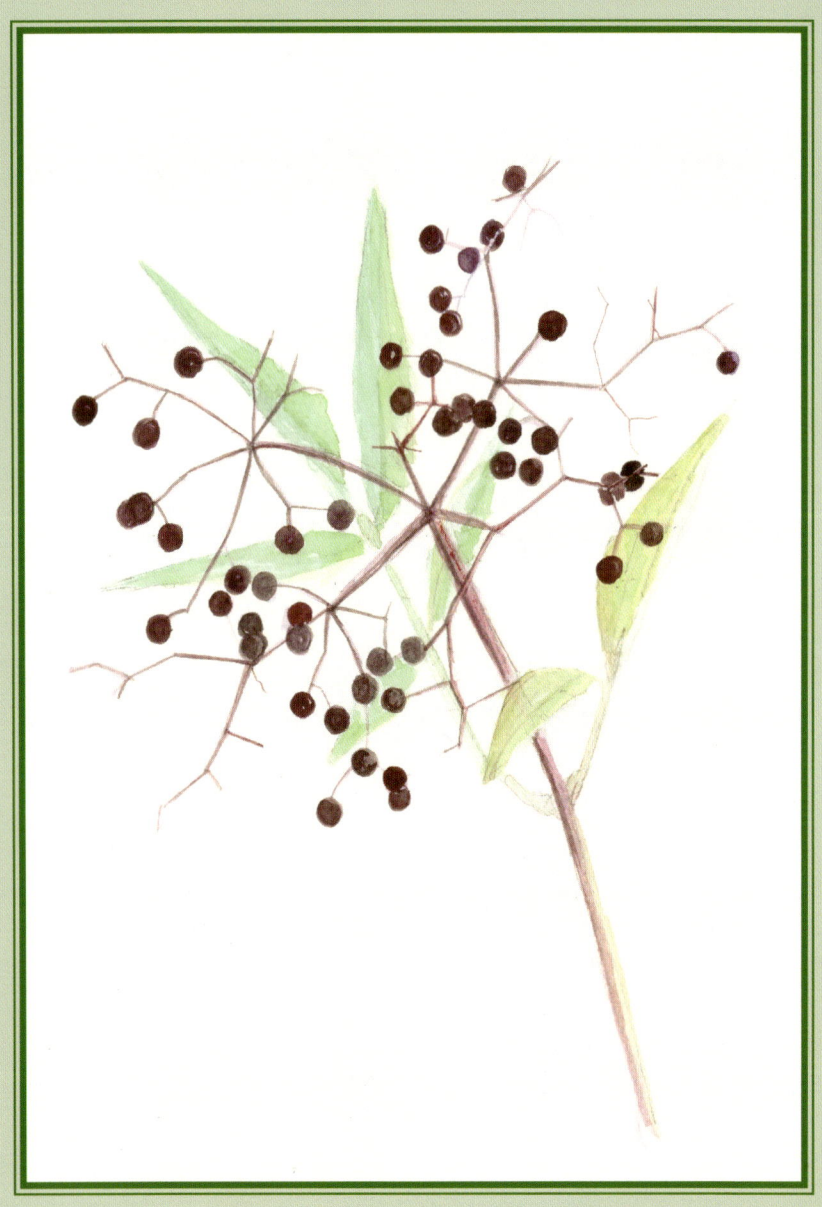

Sambucus nigra

✓ Often used to alleviate hay fever symptoms, including sneezing, runny nose, and itchy eyes, acting as an anti-catarrhal.

✓ Topically, elderflower infusions can be used as a compress for tired eyes or as a gentle skin cleanser.

Elderberry:

✓ Rich in antioxidants and vitamins, particularly Vitamin C, making it a popular immune system booster.

✓ Widely used to shorten the duration and severity of cold and flu symptoms.

✓ Possesses antiviral properties, particularly against certain strains of influenza.

✓ Can have a mild laxative effect due to its fibre content.

Spiritual benefits

The Elder is strongly associated with the feminine archetype of the 'Crone' or the 'Elder Mother' (known as *'Hylde-moer'* in Norse and Germanic folklore). This energy embodies wisdom, intuition, healing, and the cyclical nature of life, death and rebirth. It represents the deep, nurturing wisdom that comes with age and experience.

Its association with water also links it to emotions, intuition, purification and the subconscious. Water is fluid and adaptable, much like the Elder's ability to thrive in various conditions, and purifying – hence, its historical use in cleansing rituals. It also connects to the watery realms of dreams and the Otherworld.

Use for:

– Protection & warding

One of the most common associations of Elder is that of protection. It was widely planted near homes and barns in Europe, including in my home town of Upper Basildon, Berkshire, to ward off evil spirits, witches, lightning, and negative influences. Sprigs were hung over doors and windows, and carried as amulets.

– Healing & transformation

Beyond its physical medicinal properties, the Elder's subtle energy is linked to profound healing, both physical and emotional. It's believed to help release old patterns, emotional congestion, and deeply rooted fears. Its association with death and rebirth cycles also speaks to its power in guiding transformation, helping individuals to shed what no longer serves them and embrace renewal.

Associated chakras

Throat chakra: The pale, delicate flowers are linked to clarity of expression and communication, not just spoken words, but also expressing one's authentic self. This can relate to the clearing of respiratory passages, allowing for clearer breath and thus, clearer sound and thought.

Third Eye chakra: Elderflower's subtle energy can facilitate intuition, psychic awareness and connection to higher wisdom. It's said to help clear mental fog and enhance inner vision, making it beneficial for meditation and dream work. Its delicate, ethereal quality supports this connection to less tangible realms.

Root chakra: The deep, dark berries strongly resonate with grounding, protection and vital life force. Just as elderberries bolster physical immunity, they also strengthen one's energetic boundaries, providing a sense of safety and resilience. This connection helps to root one firmly in the physical world while exploring spiritual dimensions.

Sacral chakra: Elderberry's connection to vitality, creativity and the cycles of nature also links it to the Sacral chakra. It supports emotional well-being, healthy boundaries in relationships, and a flow of creative energy. The abundance of the berries themselves speaks to fertility and life's generative forces.

Tamara's Tales: Elder plant

As I write this entry, on a bright but wet afternoon in Devon at the home of my good friend and illustrator Jo Thomas, I can see two stunning 'black beauty' Elder trees, which were both grown from cuttings. I tend to use the berries more often than the flowers, to provide support against the inevitable outbreaks of flu, coughs colds and general cold 'malaise' we experience during the winter months.

The recipe below I make every year from the wonderful berries from the gorgeous elders that grow so abundantly along the fields and hedgerows of Berkshire and South Oxfordshire.

Recipe: Elderberry syrup

This recipe should taste deliciously berry-ish and spicy with the cloves, bay and cinnamon. Take a good couple of teaspoonfuls per day, and at night when you feel you need it, to relieve hay fever and cold symptoms.

What you'll need:

- 5/6 kg of elderberries washed and stripped of their stems
- 1 large, fist-sized root of fresh ginger, or several small ones, chopped
- 20 cloves
- Good shake of freshly grated nutmeg
- 5 sticks of cinnamon
- Half a pint of orange juice and the peel
- 10 freshly picked large bay leaves
- Water to fully cover
- Local honey to taste (I tend to use about five heaped tablespoons)

Method:

1. Strip the berries from the stems with a fork.
2. Once they are stripped and well washed, put them into a large boiling pot together with all the other ingredients.
3. Bring the pan up to a boil and then simmer gently for up to one hour, checking and adding a touch of water if needed.
4. Taste for sweetness and if too sharp, add more honey.
5. Let the beautiful, deep purple liquid cool off and then strain into a big muslin cloth suspended over another pot or large bowl. This could take some time as you will probably need to squeeze all the lovely juice out.

6. Place in the fridge and when fully cool, decant into clean, sterilised bottles.

Storage
I tend to keep my elderberry syrup in the fridge.

Eucalyptus

Eucalyptus oil is used medicinally as a decongestant for colds and coughs, and for its anti-inflammatory properties, to ease sore muscles.

Latin Name: *Eucalyptus globulus*

Folk Names: Blue gum, Southern Blue gum, Tasmanian Blue gum

Places of origin
Native to southeastern Australia and Tasmania.

Description
The Tasmanian blue gum tree, or *Eucalyptus globulus*, can grow exceedingly tall, and is happily naturalised all over the world.

Its bark formation is intrinsically beautiful, as it sheds perpetually: the young tree's smooth, pale blue-grey skin gives way to a vibrant jigsaw as it matures – long, strongly aromatic ribbons of reddish-browning bark peel away to reveal the creamy-yellow trunk and multi-coloured canvas of the new bark beneath.

This ever-changing portrait of striking, layered textures and shifting colours is a living testament to nature's cycle of growth and transformation.

Medicinal uses
✓ Highly regarded for its strong decongestant, expectorant and antiseptic properties.

✓ Widely used for respiratory conditions such as colds, flu, coughs, bronchitis and sinusitis to clear airways and relieve congestion.

✓ Also has analgesic and anti-inflammatory effects, useful for muscle aches and pains.

✓ Often used topically or through inhalation.

Spiritual benefits

Cleansing, invigorating, clarifying, protective, stimulating.

Associated with purification, mental clarity and fresh beginnings.

Associated chakras

Throat chakra: Primarily associated with this chakra due to its clearing effect on the respiratory system and facilitation of clear expression.

Third Eye chakra: Resonates with the Third Eye, thanks to its ability to promote mental focus and clear-thinking.

Tamara's Tales: Eucalyptus

Eucalyptus' medicinal benefits are powerful: a simple inhalation of a few drops of essential oil on a tissue can clear congested nasal pathways and release mucus from the bronchioles, giving significant relief during the cold and flu season.

When combined with menthol, rosemary and citrus lime, it can focus the mind and increase alertness, clearing the dulled mental acuity often brought about by symptoms of colds and flu.

I'm never without a bottle of eucalyptus essential oil in the winter months, and my students and colleagues alike have quickly learnt to make good use of this simple, desk-top herbal medication.

The recipe I've included is called Focus. It's a synergetic essential oil blend created to clear the mind and sharpen the senses – very useful for that mid-afternoon slump, or to encourage an early morning rise.

Recipe: Focus (10 ml blended oil)

This blend is for inhalation and use in an electronic water vapour diffuser

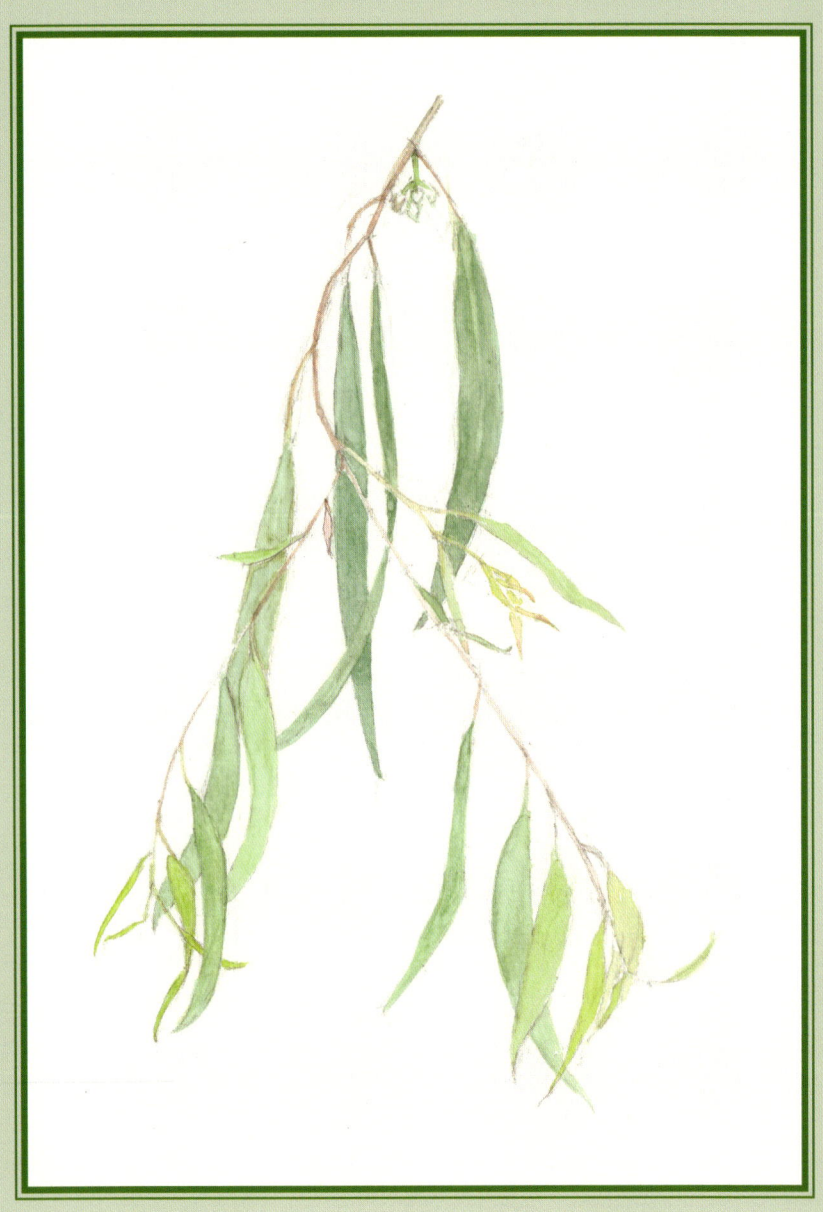

Eucalyptus globulus

– simply add a few drops to a tissue and inhale, taking care not to touch eyes, nose or mouth with the neat essential oil.

Alternatively, add to your diffuser and breathe deeply as the air is suffused with the blend, helping you to wake up and get on with your day.

What you'll need:

Pure essential oils (measure carefully):

- 1 ml (approx. 20 drops) of peppermint/spearmint essential oil
  Peppermint or spearmint essential oil has invigorating properties that stimulate the mind, increase alertness, and enhance cognitive function. It helps to clear mental fog and promote clarity of thought.
- 3 ml (approx. 60 drops) of eucalyptus essential oil
  This has a refreshing and clarifying scent that can help to clear the mind and promote mental focus. It also has stimulating properties that can boost energy levels and promote alertness.
- 1.5 ml (approx. 30 drops) of rosemary essential oil
  Renowned for its ability to improve memory, concentration, and cognitive performance, rosemary essential oil has a stimulating aroma that can enhance mental clarity and focus.
- 1.5 ml (approx. 30 drops) of lime essential oil
  Adds a bright and citrusy scent to the blend, which helps to uplift the mood and invigorate the senses. It provides a refreshing burst of energy and can help to promote mental alertness.

Method:

1. Pour the oils into a 20 ml glass measuring beaker.
2. Stir the synergetic mix together using a glass rod, and swirl the jar to ensure it's all blended.
3. Carefully pipette into a sanitised, 10 ml dark glass essential oil dropping bottle.
4. Fix on the dropper top and label.

Storage & expiry

Store in a cool, dark spot. Use within two years.

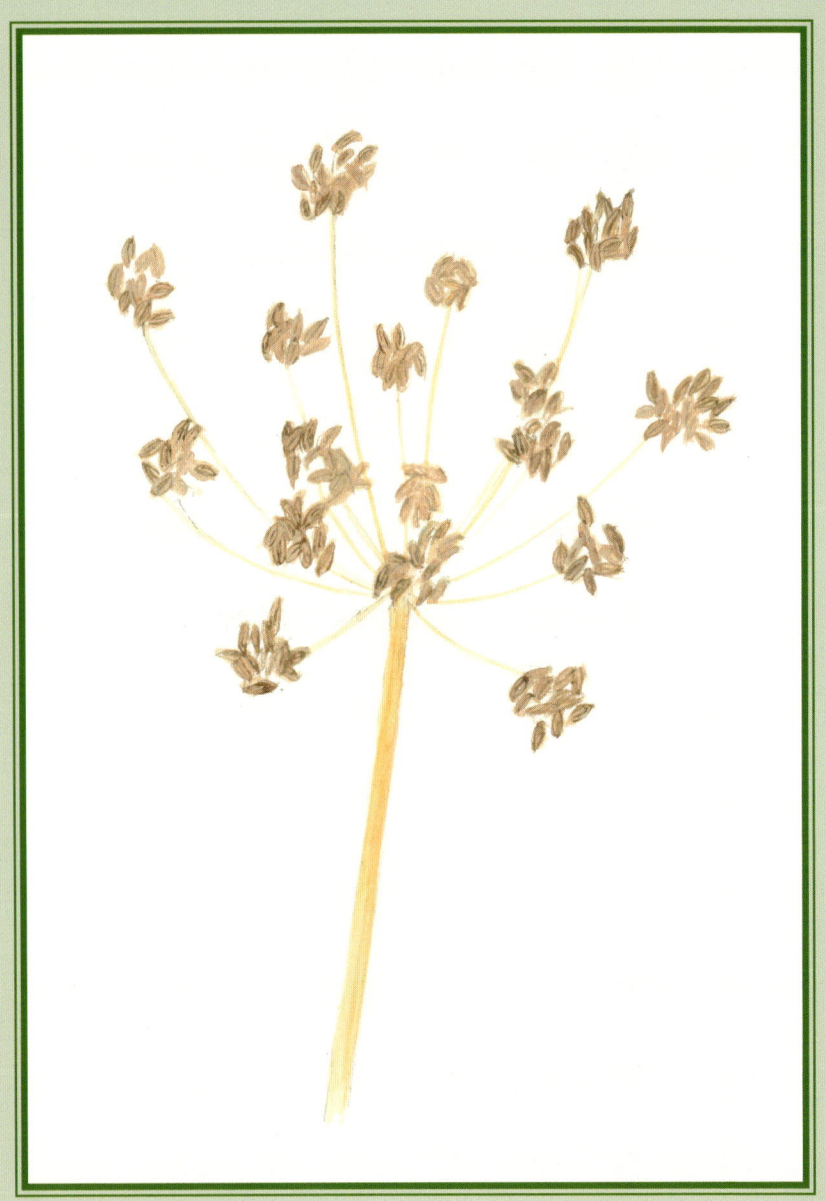

Foeniculum vulgare

Fennel

The benefits of fennel have been known for millennia. Its anti-inflammatory and tummy-settling properties make it the perfect staple for your herbal plant collection.

Latin name: *Foeniculum vulgare*

Folk names: Sweet fennel, Wild fennel, Florence fennel, finocchio, saffron

Places of origin

Native to the Mediterranean region, with a long history of cultivation throughout Europe, Asia and North America.

Description

Fennel has had a majestic presence across the European landscape since ancient times. Its sylph-like beauty lies not only in its lengthy and graceful branched fronds, which are topped abundantly with umbelled summer-yellow florets and filigree leaflets, but also its milky-white and pale green edible bulb. Its magnificently seeded flower heads can reach up to 1.5 metres or more.

The seeds of the fennel have a well-documented repertoire of medicinal uses dating back to entries on Mycenaean tablets more than 5,000 years ago. The plant is so popular in Greece that its Greek name, *'Maratho'*, was given in antiquity to a vast number of cities and settlements, including Marathon, in Attica.

Medicinal uses

- ✓ Traditionally used to aid digestion, with fennel seed & fennel seed oil shown to offer significant anti-inflammatory properties:
  - – Helping soothe swelling & irritation in gastrointestinal tract to reduce bloating, releasing trapped wind.
  - – Said to help relax muscles of gastrointestinal tract, relieving bloating & improving digestion thanks to a chemical called anethole.

– Can be very helpful for IBS and to support motility.

✓ Containing antifungal and antibacterial properties, fennel seeds have an antimicrobial function.

✓ Known as a 'galactagogue', it can help increase milk production in lactating mothers.

✓ Cold-pressed fennel seed carrier oil has phytoestrogenic actions, often used to support the female cycle to help with symptoms of PMT and menopause.

Note: Fennel essential oil is extremely potent and should not be confused with **pressed fennel seed oil**. I *do not* recommend using fennel seed essential oil unless fully trained in aromatherapy blending.

Spiritual benefits

Protective, grounding, strengthening, purifying.

Associated with courage, longevity, and clear communication. It's also believed to ward off negative energy.

Associated chakras

Solar Plexus chakra: For its digestive support and the confidence it instils.

Sacral chakra: Due to its connection with reproductive health and hormonal balance.

Tamara's Tales: Fennel

My relationship with fennel began in earnest when I began to suffer badly with Irritable Bowel Syndrome (IBS), around the time of my hysterectomy. Looking back, it was clearly a consequence of a stressful lifestyle with, as it seemed to me at the time, no way out. My gut-brain connection was in overdrive and my digestion eventually shut down.

My doctor suggested antidepressants, which I didn't want to entertain at that time. Instead, I avoided gluten, and every morning before leaving for work I started taking fennel seeds and flax soaked in warm water with the juice of half a lemon. I couldn't do breakfast as it wouldn't digest.

After a month or so, things seemed much easier, motility-wise. I kept this up for a couple of years and managed to regulate my digestion and keep my IBS at bay.

Recipe: Fennel seed tea

This recipe is the perfect tummy-settler with a powerful combination of ingredients, including peppermint and ginger.

What you'll need:

- Teapot
- 2 tablespoons dried fennel seed
- Fresh ginger, washed and chopped (no need to peel) – enough to cover the bottom of a teapot to two inches
- A good handful of freshly washed peppermint from the garden

Method:

1. Place dried fennel seed into a teapot
2. Add fresh ginger and peppermint leaves
3. Fill the pot with boiling water and leave to infuse for 10 minutes
4. Using a tea strainer, pour into mugs
5. Add a teaspoon of local organic honey to taste and sip slowly, to settle your tummy.

Frankincense

Frankincense has long been revered and used in sacred rituals to strengthen connection to the divine. Used medicinally to alleviate joint pain, support respiratory and digestive function, and to rejuvenate the skin.

Latin name: *Boswellia carterii* (the specific scientific name for the frankincense species talked about in this book; there are other *Boswellia* species that also produce frankincense resin)

Folk names: Olibanum (another common name, especially in historical and religious texts); Luban (Arabic name; widely used in the regions where it grows); Beyo (Somali name)

Places of origin

Boswellia carterii is native to the arid and semi-arid regions of Northeast Africa and the Arabian Peninsula. Its primary habitats include Somalia, Yemen and Oman.

Description

The frankincense tree is a scraggly, shrub-like plant with peeling bark, often found clinging to rocky cliffs and arid landscapes.

Its resin is collected by 'tapping': a shallow incision is made in the tree's trunk, causing a milky-white, sap-like resin to bleed out. Over several weeks, this sap hardens into tear-shaped droplets, which are then scraped from the bark. These hardened 'tears' are translucent and can range in colour from pale yellow or green, to amber.

Frankincense essential oil is a pale yellow-green liquid with a complex fragrance that's both woody and spicy, with a hint of citrus. The oil is a staple in aromatherapy and traditional medicine, for its calming properties and use in skincare.

Medicinal uses

✓ Valued for its anti-inflammatory properties historically, as well as in modern herbalism (supported by modern research), helping ease joint pain and swelling.

✓ Respiratory support: Traditionally inhaled as smoke or used in preparations for coughs, bronchitis and asthma.

✓ Skin health: An antiseptic, applied topically to help heal wounds, reduce scars and improve skin appearance.

✓ Oral health: Used in some cultures as a chewing gum for its antiseptic properties and to freshen breath.

✓ Digestive aid: Traditionally used to soothe digestive upset.

✓ Emotional and spiritual well-being: Its aromatic smoke is used to promote relaxation, focus and a sense of peace.

✓ Essential oil of frankincense is popular for its calming and grounding effects, used to slow and deepen the breath, reducing stress and promoting relaxation.

Spiritual benefits

The aroma of frankincense is deeply connected to its energetic properties and has been revered for its ability to promote spiritual connection; it's believed to facilitate a deeper connection to the divine, and enhance spiritual practices.

Associated chakras

Crown chakra: Its ability to promote spiritual connection, transcendence and a sense of unity aligns strongly with this chakra – the centre of higher consciousness and spiritual awareness.

Third Eye chakra: Frankincense's capacity to enhance mental clarity, intuition and focus resonates with the Third Eye, the centre of wisdom and inner vision.

Root chakra: It can also have a balancing effect on the Root, due to its grounding properties, helping create a stable foundation for spiritual exploration.

Tamara's Tales: Frankincense

I've often turned to frankincense to help get back on my feet and back to work after attacks of viral flu.

I mix the essential oil with eucalyptus and use it in my diffuser at night, and also soak a warmed flannel in a carrier mix of four tablespoons of jojoba/olive/sweet almond oil and five drops each of frankincense, eucalyptus and lavender essential oils, and lay it on my chest before sleeping. The oil mix penetrates the stratum corneum layer of the skin and begins to sooth the congestion and inflammation quickly.

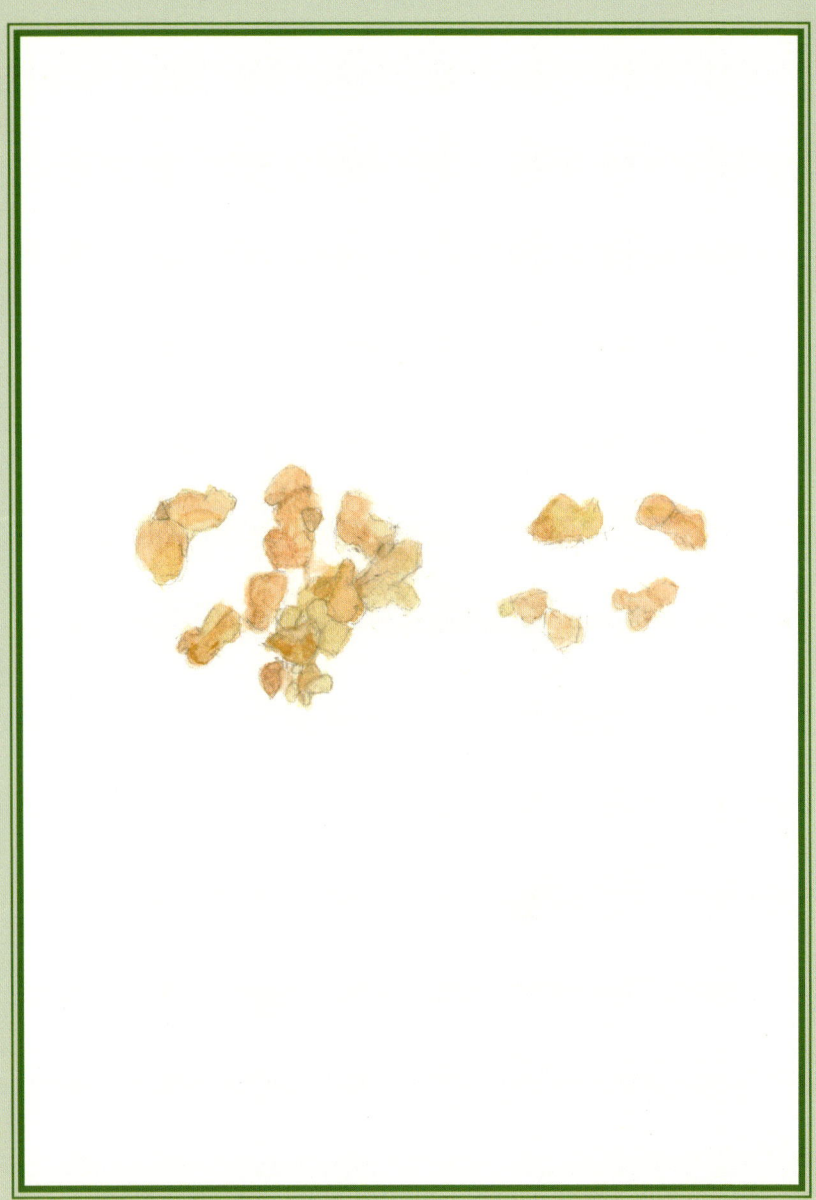

Boswellia carterii

Recipe: Frankincense night cream

A nutrient-rich, light and fluffy face cream to help rejuvenate your skin overnight.

What you'll need:

- 6 tablespoons (approx. 60 ml) base cream formulated from natural ingredients and paraben-free
- 2 tablespoons calendula-infused olive oil*
- 2 tablespoons chamomile-infused olive oil*
- 75 ml of rose/ lavender hydrosol
- 1 ml (approx. 20 drops) of frankincense essential oil**
- 2 ml (approx. 50 drops) of lavender essential oil
- 5 drops ylang ylang essential oil
- 5 drops naturally derived preservative, Benzoic acid
- 5 drops vitamin E oil

*Can be substituted with jojoba, avocado, pomegranate or sweet almond oil.

**This oil is very concentrated so don't be tempted to use more.*

Method:

1. Combine the base cream and infused oils together in a 500 ml glass measuring beaker using a glass rod stirrer.
2. Drizzle in the hydrosol, benzoic acid and vitamin E oil
3. Hand blend till creamy and light
4. Add the synergetic mix of essential oils and blend again
5. Pour, scrape or pipe into one or two 100 ml sanitised dark glass cosmetics jars
6. Use with joy at night for a soothing, rejuvenating face cream.

Storage & expiry

Store in a cool, dry spot. Use within six months.

Ginger

Ginger is a treasure in the medicine chest with a long history of use, both as a culinary spice and a powerful medicine. A jewel above and below the ground, the plant has two component parts, both of which offer rich benefits, which include anti-nausea, anti-inflammatory and decongestant properties.

Latin name: *Zingiber officinale*

Folk names: Common ginger, Jamaican ginger, African ginger, Canton ginger, Black ginger, Race ginger

Places of origin

Believed to have originated in Maritime Southeast Asia, likely in the Indian subcontinent or the Malay Archipelago. Ginger has been cultivated for more than 5,000 years and is now grown in tropical climates around the world.

Description

The ginger rhizome and its tropical flower are a study in contrasts — one a gnarled anchor of spicy earth, the other a delicate bloom of fleeting beauty.

The ginger rhizome

Hidden beneath the soil, the rhizome is a thick, fleshy and highly branched underground stem. Its colour can vary, from a pale, creamy yellow to a more saturated golden hue, and even a reddish-purple in some varieties. The exterior is a light-brown, corky skin, often covered in ridges, rings and bumpy 'eyes', from which new shoots and roots emerge.

When sliced, the flesh reveals its fibrous texture, with a potent, citrusy aroma and a fiery, pungent flavour that intensifies with maturity: a storehouse of energy and medicinal warmth and vitality.

Tropical ginger flower

The ginger flower is a rare and beautiful sight in cultivation. It emerges on a short stem directly from the rhizome – a world away from the leafy stalks.

The inflorescence is a dense, cone-shaped spike from which the delicate flowers emerge. Each flower is a fragile, short-lived bloom with pale yellow-to-greenish petals and a striking purple-spotted lip. This 'lip' is a modified petal that serves as a landing platform for pollinators.

The entire flower head is nestled among overlapping, yellowish-green bracts, creating a mosaic of subtle, tropical colours. This bloom is a fleeting and elegant spectacle; a gentle flourish from a plant renowned for its powerful, earthy core.

Medicinal uses

A key medicinal herb for millennia, ginger's primary active compounds are gingerols and shogaols, which give it its pungent flavour and therapeutic effects.

Historical uses

Ginger was a highly valued commodity along the ancient Silk Road trade routes.

In both Ayurvedic and TCM, ginger has been a cornerstone herb for thousands of years. It was used to treat digestive disorders, nausea, and to warm the body during cold and flu season. The philosopher Confucius was said to eat ginger with every meal.

The Greeks and Romans imported ginger from the East and used it for its medicinal properties, particularly for its digestive benefits, and the physician Dioscorides documented its use for indigestion and as an antidote to poisons.

In Europe, Ginger was a popular spice and medicine, valued especially for its ability to preserve meat and for its warming qualities. It was highly prized and used to ward off the plague and other illnesses.

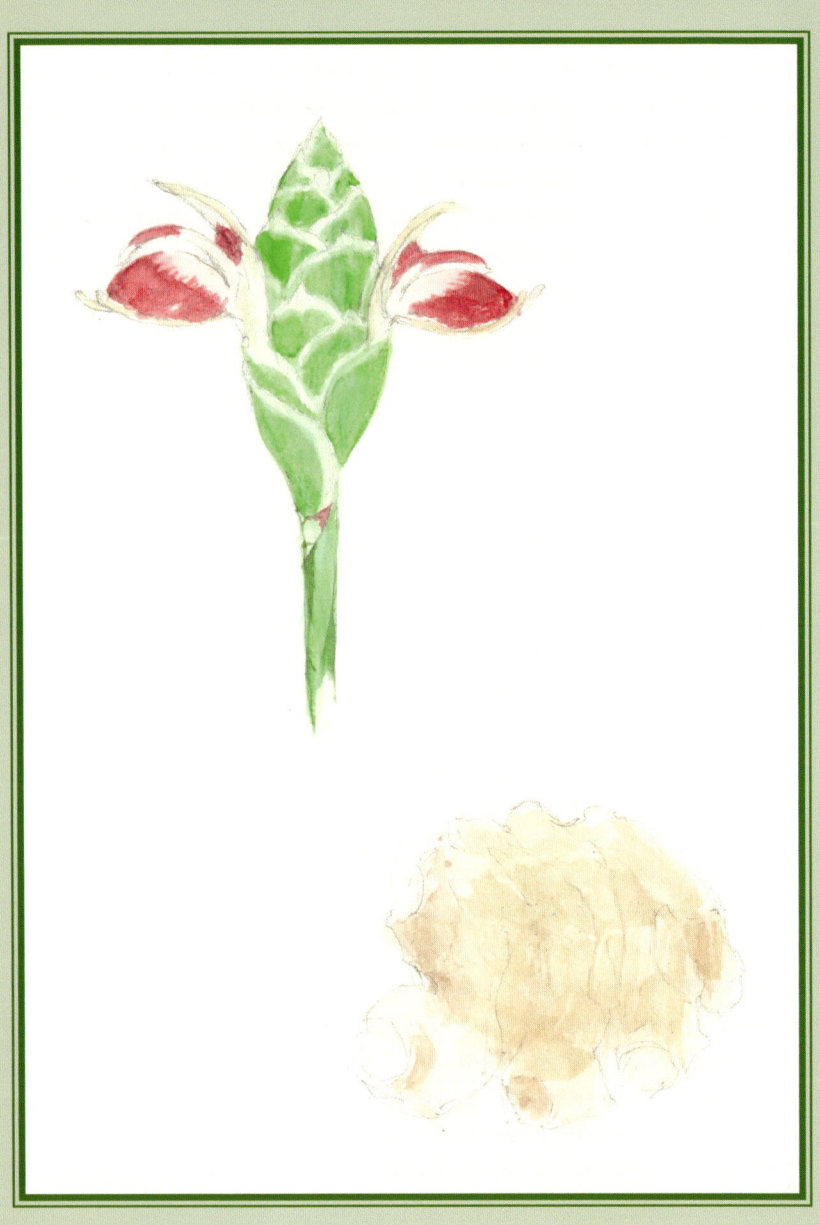

Zingiber officinale

Current uses

- ✓ Most famous for its potent anti-emetic (anti-nausea) and carminative (anti-gas) properties.

- ✓ Stimulates saliva and bile production, helping food move more smoothly through the digestive tract. The active compounds relax the smooth muscles in the gut, helping prevent spasms and discomfort. This makes ginger highly effective for indigestion, bloating and gas.

- ✓ Ginger's powerful anti-nausea effects are well-documented. Widely used to prevent and treat motion sickness, morning sickness during pregnancy and nausea caused by chemotherapy. Its active compounds interact with serotonin receptors in the gut and brain, which are a major pathway for nausea signals.

- ✓ Gingerols are potent anti-inflammatory agents that can inhibit the production of pro-inflammatory compounds in the body. This makes ginger beneficial for relieving pain and inflammation associated with conditions such as osteoarthritis and muscle soreness.

- ✓ Immune support: Traditionally used to warm the body and promote sweating (diaphoretic), ginger is a popular remedy for colds and flu. It can help clear congestion and soothe a sore throat, with its warming nature supporting the body's natural fever response.

Spiritual benefits

Associated with a strong, fiery and active masculine energy. This relates to ginger's warming, stimulating and purifying effects on both the physical body and the spirit – it embodies a dynamic force that can cut through stagnation and lethargy.

Its signature pungent taste and heat link it directly to the element of Fire, representing passion, purification, transformation and vitality. Ginger's fiery nature helps to 'burn away' what no longer serves, both physically and energetically.

Associated chakras

Root chakra: The deep-rooted rhizome and its warming energy ground and stabilise the physical body. It's excellent for strengthening your connection to the earth, and for building a sense of security and resilience.

Ginger can help individuals feel more present and embodied.

Sacral chakra: Ginger's stimulating, fiery energy resonates with this chakra, as the centre of creativity, passion and vitality. It can help ignite creative sparks, enhance libido, and bring a sense of zest and enthusiasm to life.

Tamara's Tales: Ginger

I witnessed a huge crop of these beautiful blooms growing in Jamaica down a gully when my son was only three, and was utterly transfixed.

My recipe's a simple ginger tea, which my daughter loves to make. We use it for colds, cough, flu and upset tummy.

Recipe: Jamaican ginger tea

What you'll need:

- 2/3 inches fresh ginger root, peeled and grated
- 5 black peppercorns
- 1 sprig fresh thyme
- 2 cloves
- 1 fresh bay leaf
- Juice of half a lemon
- Organic local honey to taste
- 3/4 pint of water

Method:

1. Place all ingredients in a pan and bring to the boil.
2. Simmer for 15 - 20 minutes to make a decoction (strong tea).
3. It should be a milky colour with a strong ginger taste.
4. Allow to cool, strain and sip gently.

Lavender

Lavender is renowned for its aromatic qualities, as well as its ability to bring a moment of calm on inhalation. This beautiful botanical can also be used to treat minor skin irritation, thanks to its antiseptic properties, and is also used for its analgesic effects on aching muscles.

Latin name: *Lavandula angustifolia* (common lavender species)

Folk names: True lavender, English lavender, Garden lavender, Common lavender

Places of origin

Native to the Mediterranean region, the Middle East and India.

Description

Beyond the most familiar fields of purple haze, the lavender plant is a quiet marvel of understated beauty and robust fragrance, with a spectrum of varieties that reach far beyond a single hue.

Her flowers, clustered on slender spikes, are not only purple, but can be found in shades of white, pink and even a deep, moody violet – each, a tiny bell or whorl holding precious essential oil to calm the spirit.

The leaves contribute to lavender's subtle charm and also release oil; they are typically a silvery-green or grey, are slim and lance-like, sometimes velvety to the touch, and hold a delicate, resinous aroma even before the blooms unfurl, hinting at the powerful essence to come.

Together, these elements form a hardy, aromatic plant that stands as a testament to nature's diverse and aromatic artistry.

Medicinal uses

- ✓ Lavender is widely known for its calming, anxiolytic and sedative properties.
- ✓ Used to reduce stress, anxiety and insomnia, and to promote relaxation.

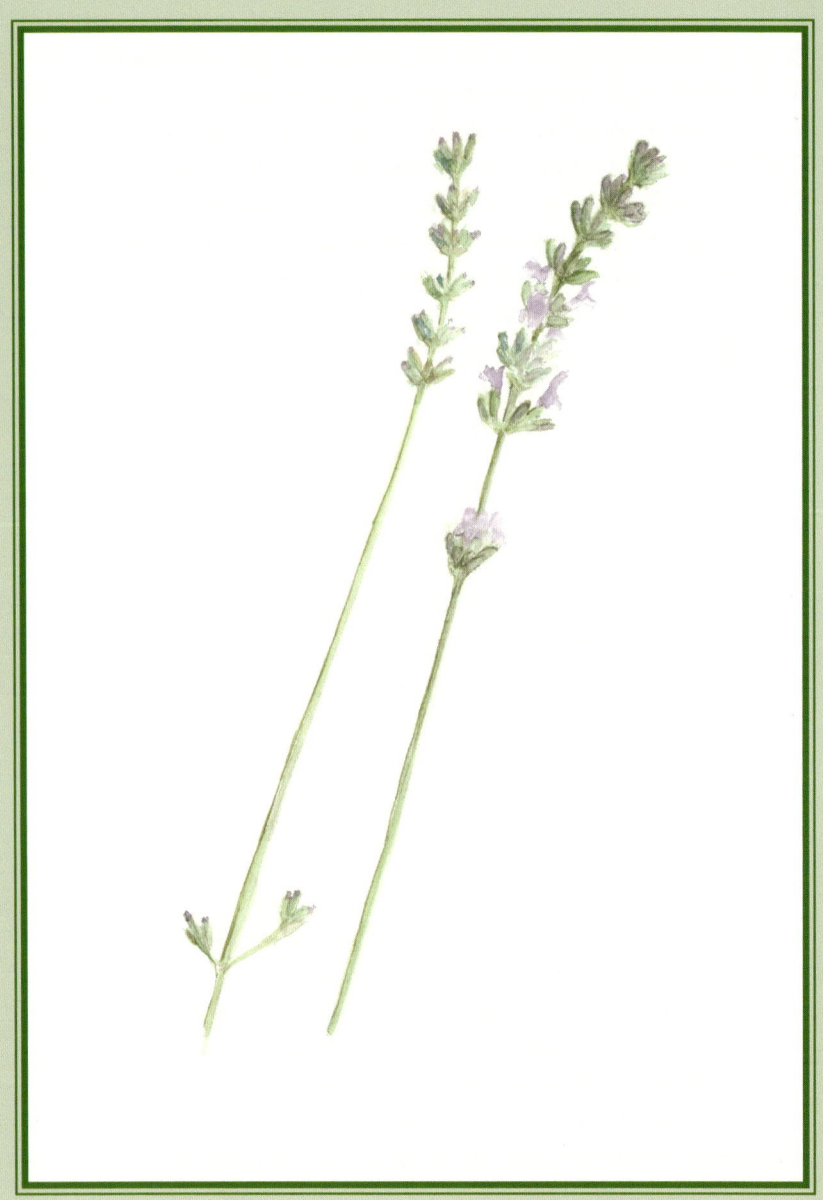

Lavandula angustifolia

✓ Known to have analgesic, anti-inflammatory and antiseptic properties, making lavender useful for headaches, muscle aches, minor burns and skin irritations.

Spiritual benefits

Calming, purifying, balancing, soothing, peaceful.

Associated with tranquillity, spiritual cleansing and emotional stability.

Associated chakras

Third Eye chakra: Known for calming the mind and enhancing intuition.

Crown chakra: Opens connection to spiritual peace and higher consciousness.

Throat chakra: Has a soothing effect this chakra, due to her calming influence on communication.

Tamara's Tales: Lavender

In my eyes, lavender's the undisputed 'Queen of Herbs'. In the early days of motherhood, I discovered that lavender essential oil not only calmed me down and sent me gently to sleep, but did the same for my wonderful children, too. It was also brilliant for cuts, grazes, stings, bites and headaches.

A light dab with a drop of lavender oil and we all felt better...immeasurably! From that moment, I was never without a bottle or two in my bag, in the bathroom and on my bedside table.

I began growing lavender myself, and by the time I settled in Greece some 20 years later, I set about creating large terraces of Greek lavandin: a potent hybrid with long, deeply aromatic flower heads yielding incredibly potent essential oil, and attracting hundreds of happy pollinators.

I began experimenting, progressing from a glass steam distillation condenser with a one-litre capacity, to five litres and eventually, a 35-litre unit so I could distil all the beautiful essential oils and create the hydrosol – the wonderful, perfumed water left over after distillation. Through many a trial and error, I created a line of candles, soaps, balms, sprays, synergetic blends, face and body creams, and bath oils.

The roots of my passion with herbs stems from my early experiences with the healing potential of lavender as a pain-relieving, anti-inflammatory, sedative plant for family use and self-care. Now, writing this story in Greece all those years later, less than five miles away from my original lavender terraces, I can still smell their sweet perfume, mingled with wild oregano on the breeze…

Recipe: Lavender skin balm

A gentle, aromatic balm that's a wonderful addition to any self-care routine. When combined with nourishing oils and beeswax, this lavender balm creates a powerful ally for soothing irritated skin, promoting minor wound healing, and simply offering a moment of aromatic tranquillity.

What you'll need:

- 8 tablespoons (approx. 120 ml) lavender-infused base oil (preferably olive oil)
- 1 tablespoon (8g) organic beeswax pellets
- 4 tablespoons (approx. 60 ml) shea butter (refined or unrefined)
- 2 ml (approx. 40 drops) lavender essential oil (*Lavandula angustifolia*)
- 6 drops vitamin E oil (optional)

Method:

1. Combine base oil, beeswax and shea butter in a bain marie and melt, stirring occasionally over gentle heat.

> **Tam's tip**
> *Try taking off the heat and adding the shea butter last – this seems to help avoid a grainy texture when the mixture sets.*

2. When fully combined and cooler, add the lavender essential oil and vitamin E.
3. Next, carefully pour the liquid balm into a pouring jug and decant into clean, small shallow tins or glass cosmetic jars.

4. Allow the balm to cool completely at room temperature until it solidifies. This may take a few hours. Try not to be tempted to touch the surface, as this dents the smooth finish!

5. Once solid, secure the lids.

Storage & expiry

Store in a cool, dark place and use within one year.

Testimonial

'I was recommended Tamara's products through a friend. As someone who struggles to switch off at night, I was looking for a natural remedy that would help me relax and unwind. Tamara's consultation was amazing, she really listened to what I wanted/needed and was able to create a bespoke selection of natural sleep and pain relief remedies. I highly recommend her products, they worked and I haven't looked back since!'

Sophie Cadman

Lemon balm

Lemon balm is a versatile plant with powerful properties that can support our health medicinally and emotionally, such as uplifting your mood and aiding digestion.

Latin name: *Melissa officinalis*

Folk names: Balm, common balm, balm mint, garden balm, sweet balm, Melissa

Places of origin

Native to the temperate zone, the Mediterranean region and Western Asia.

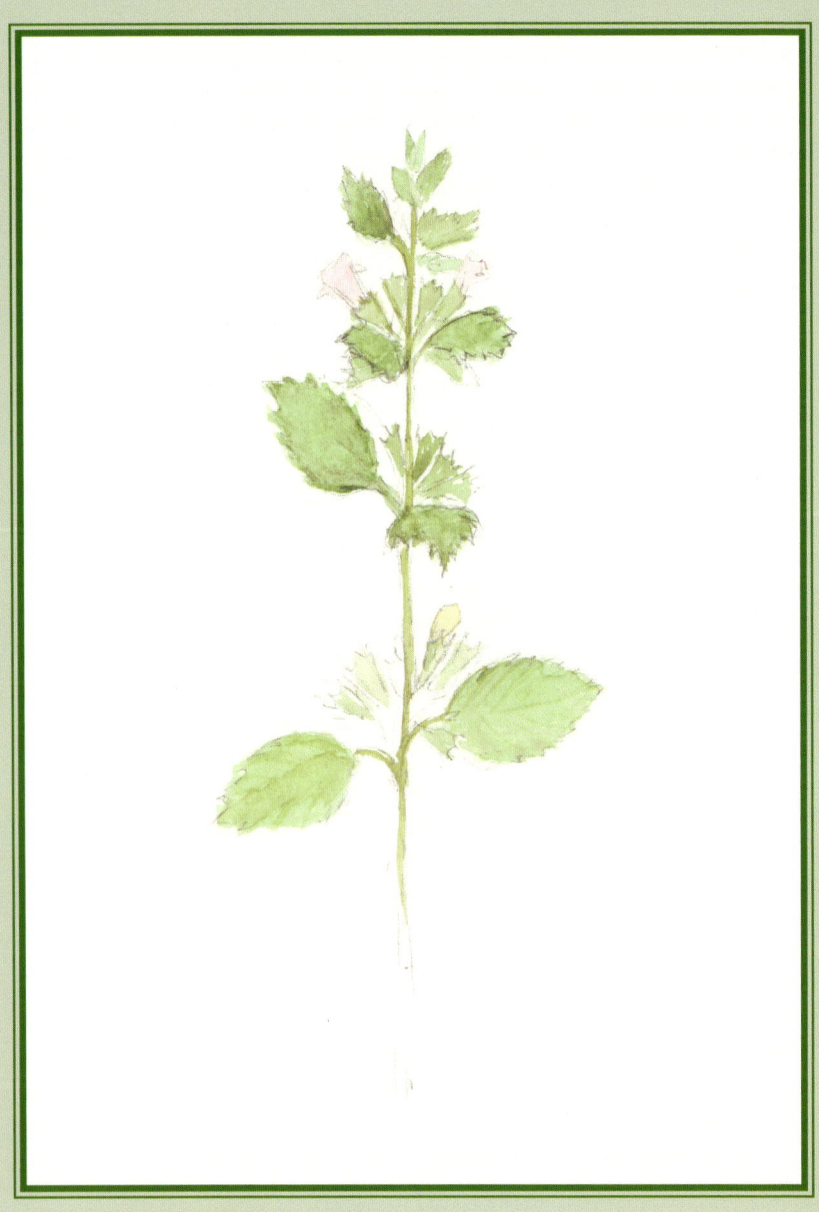

Melissa officinalis

Description

Lemon balm is a common perennial herb with heart-shaped, veined, and slightly hairy leaves, looking a bit like nettles; you'll very probably have some growing in your garden. Gentle and unassuming, with a bushy yet graceful growth, it happily takes root in cultivation and in the wild.

Also known as 'Melissa', which comes from the Greek word *'melios'*, meaning honey, its scent is gorgeous: honeyed, sweet and 'lemony', and has an immediate effect on the emotions. It was used historically by beekeepers, who would rub the leaves of the lemon balm around the hives to keep the bees close by.

The 17th-century botanist Culpepper said that lemon balm 'causeth the mind and heart to become merry and driveth away all troublesome cares and thoughts'.

Medicinal uses

✓ Renowned for its calming and mood-lifting properties.

✓ Used to reduce stress and anxiety, and improve sleep.

✓ Helps soothe digestive issues.

✓ Relieve headaches.

✓ Has antiviral properties, particularly against the herpes simplex virus.

Spiritual benefits

Calming, uplifting, soothing, joyful, comforting, heart-opening.

Associated with emotional healing, peace, and gentle joy.

Associated chakras

Heart chakra: Has the ability to soothe emotional distress and open the heart.

Solar Plexus chakra: For its calming effect on nervous digestion and gently uplifting energy.

Tamara's Tales: Lemon balm

Lemon balm's one of my favourite garden plants. It can be used gently by picking the fresh leaves for teas or simply rubbing between the hands and inhaling when you're in the garden – or more powerfully via the essential oil, through inhalation, vapour or topical application.

I've used lemon balm in every way conceivable, and my recipe incorporates the essential oil into a topical skin balm, for emotional support as well as skin care. I first made this balm in Greece, to support a bereaved guest who'd come to try and work through her feelings of loss and grief. I'd grown huge swathes of lemon balm in my herbal gardens and we experimented in my workshop with the home-distilled essential oil, creating creamy concoctions, balms and soaps using lemon balm as a key ingredient.

Recipe: Nurture balm

This balm is intended to support emotional balance when emotions feel raw – providing a nervine tonic and uplifting the mood, as well as nourishing the skin.

What you'll need:

- 2 tablespoons chamomile-infused oil/jojoba
- 2 tablespoons cocoa butter
- 1 tablespoon St John's wort balsam/pomegranate oil
- 1 tablespoon evening primrose oil/borage (starflower oil)
- 2 tablespoons shea butter
- 1 tablespoon beeswax pellets
- 0.5 ml (10 drops) Melissa
- 1.5 ml (30 drops) lavender
- 0.5 ml (10 drops) clary sage
- 0.5 ml (10 drops) lemon verbena
- 0.5 ml (10 drops) neroli
- 50 ml rose hydrosol
- 3 drops vitamin E
- 2 drops Benzoic acid preservative

Method:

1. Gently melt together the wax, oils and butters in a bain marie.
2. Allow to cool but still remain liquid.
3. Pour into a room-temperature glass mixing bowl and add the essential oil blend.
4. Whisk together using a small, hand-held blender on the lowest setting.
5. Carefully drizzle in the rose hydrosol and blend until you get a fluffy, thickened emulsion.
6. Carefully pour, spoon and scrape the mixture into two sterilised cosmetics jars or containers.
7. Leave to fully cool.
8. Gently warm in the hands before using as a massage balm for body, feet, temples and tummy, or as an after-bath/shower body balm to gently support the psyche during emotional times.

Storage & expiry

Store in a cool dry spot. Use within six months.

Orange tree

The orange tree comes in many variations, each offering bountiful fruits prized for their oils and beneficial properties. This plant profile focuses on oils from the bitter orange and sweet orange tree, with therapeutic uses ranging from supporting shock to soothing the digestion and uplifting the spirits.

Folk names: Sweet orange, China orange, Navel orange

Places of origin

Native to Southeast Asia, specifically China, and has been cultivated for thousands of years. It was brought to the Mediterranean by traders and is now grown in warm climates all over the world.

Description

Sweet orange tree
Latin name: *Citrus sinensis*

The sweet orange tree is a symbol of simple, sun-drenched happiness. Its bright fruit and glossy, deep green leaves hold a familiar, pure sweetness and aroma. Both the sweet and bitter orange trees are evergreen, so their leaves stay vibrant all year round.

Essential oil derivative:

Sweet orange
Plant part: Distilled or pressed from the peel of the ripe fruit.

Bitter orange tree
Latin name: *Citrus aurantium*

The bitter orange tree is more complex. Its sharp thorns and sour fruit belie the intense, beautiful fragrance of its flowers and leaves, which are the source of neroli and petitgrain essential oils. It's a tree of contrasts, offering a sophisticated and layered scent rather than just a simple sweetness.

Essential oil derivative:

Petitgrain
Plant part: Distilled from the leaves and twigs.

Neroli
Plant part: Oil is stored in the fragrant, waxy, white flowers and gathered by steam distillation.

Medicinal uses

- ✓ Orange tree fruit is a well-known source of vitamin C, supporting the immune system.
- ✓ Orange peel, leaves and flowers are used in traditional medicine for their calming, digestive and antiseptic properties.

✓ The fruit and leaves have been used historically to soothe stomach issues and promote relaxation.

(Aromatherapy)

✓ Sweet orange

A cheerful and uplifting oil, sweet orange is widely used to reduce stress, anxiety and feelings of depression. It's known to promote feelings of happiness and a sense of calm.

Also used in household cleaners for its antibacterial properties and pleasant aroma.

✓ Petitgrain

This oil is known for its calming and balancing properties. It's often used to alleviate nervous tension, stress and insomnia, and to promote a sense of emotional clarity and self-acceptance. It has a fresh, woody-floral scent with a citrus undertone.

✓ Neroli

A highly prized essential oil, neroli is one of the most effective oils for treating anxiety, shock, and panic. Its delicate, floral aroma is deeply calming, uplifting the spirit while also acting as a sedative. Also a popular ingredient in skincare for its rejuvenating properties.

Spiritual benefits

Joy, abundance, creativity and purification.

The orange tree is associated with a bright, uplifting energy that promotes happiness and a positive outlook, and is believed to bring warmth and light, helping dispel gloom and stagnation. Its presence is believed to attract good fortune and prosperity.

Associated chakras

Sweet orange essential oil

Sacral chakra: For creativity, pleasure, emotion, and passion. Sweet orange is believed to help release emotional blockages, inspire joy and promote a sense of creative flow.

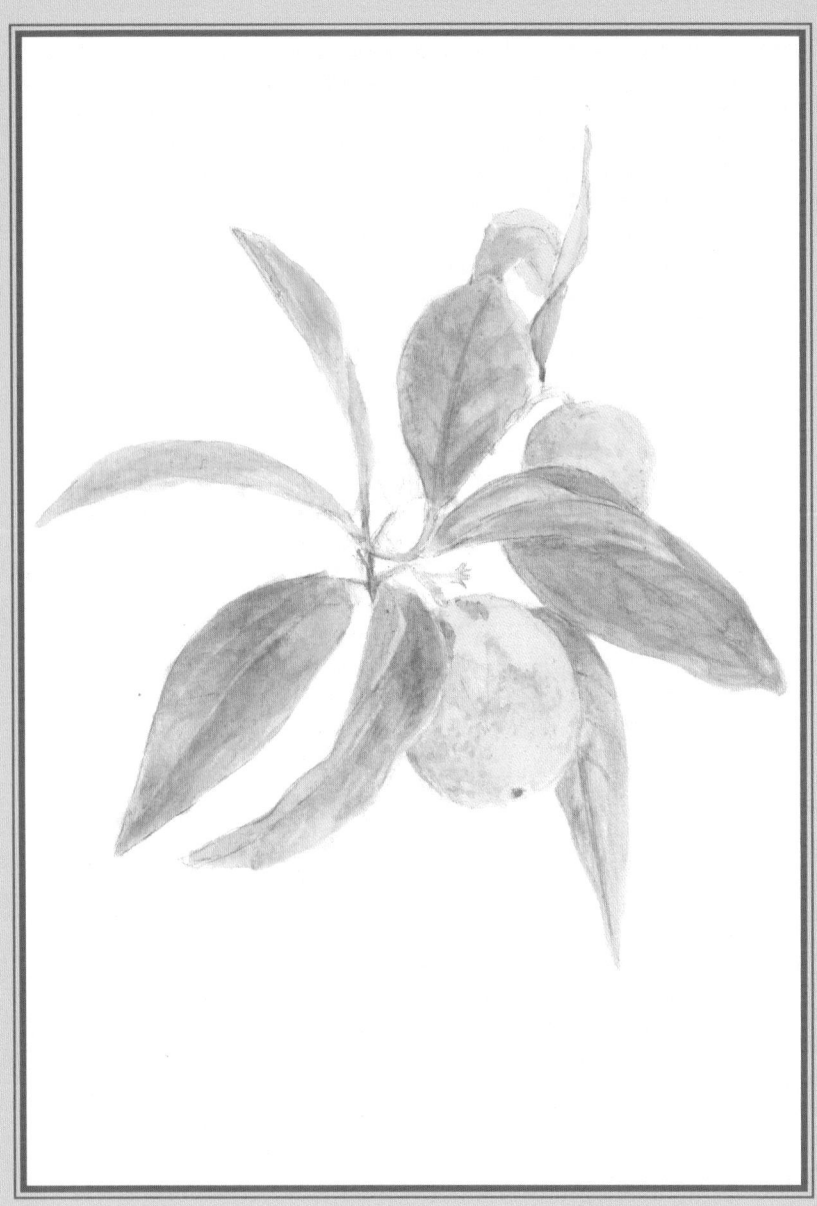

Citrus aurantium

Neroli essential oil

Crown chakra: Neroli's high-vibrational scent fosters a spiritual connection, encouraging self-awareness and supporting meditation.

Heart chakra: It has the ability to soothe emotional wounds, open the heart to love, and calm feelings of anxiety and grief.

Petitgrain essential oil

Solar Plexus chakra: Boosts personal power, self-esteem and confidence. Petitgrain's calming and clarifying properties are thought to help release feelings of fear and stress, promoting a sense of inner peace and grounding.

Tamara's Tales: Orange tree

The orange, for most of us in the UK, evokes the festive season. I love to stud oranges with cloves and stick on star anise, and tie cinnamon rolls with ribboned bows to festoon the conservatory with aromatic pomanders at Christmas time. For me, the aromas waft delicious memories of contentment and carols.

In Greece, the oranges fully ripen in December, swelling plumply in the autumn with the welcome rain. Making marmalade was one of my favourite pastimes during my great Greek adventure. We had five fruitful trees and an additional two lemon trees, and our friends had another six down at the bottom of the olive grove.

First job: pick and carry the heavy fruit in wheelbarrows up to the kitchen. Second job: peel and pith several hundred fruit!

I bought a huge, steel boiling pan and used a gigantic wooden spoon for making my marmalade. The three ingredients were oranges, lemons and raw cane sugar. I had two juicers and a peeler, and by the time I finished, the entire kitchen was covered in citrus and smelt heavenly.

Jars in trays were sanitised in the oven, and pectin produced by boiling lemon peels, pith and seeds in a muslin bag with the juice fruit and sugar for several hours on end. The process took a couple of days, at least, with lots of testing for the correct jelly-like consistency.

But after a few practice runs, I could reliably produce over 100 jars of absolutely delicious orange and lemon marmalade for friends, family and for sale. To this day, we all agree that the marmalade I made in Greece from the oranges in the grove was the best-tasting marmalade of our lives!

The recipe below is not to eat, though the scent is delicious; it's a recipe for a super-indulgent, relaxing and skin-loving bath oil.

Recipe: Extraordinary bath oil

This recipe uses an organic almond oil based, dispersible bath oil which enables the essential oils to disperse safely and be absorbed through the skin with maximum benefit. You only need a couple of capfuls, as the synergistic mix is intense – the tiny molecules of the essentials oil can enter the skin through the pores and most of your body will be immersed in the water, making the overall effect far stronger.

Makes one litre.

What you'll need:

- 850 ml dispersible bath oil*
- 1 tablespoon (approx. 45 ml) avocado oil
- 2 tablespoons (approx. 30 ml) chamomile-infused olive oil
- 2 tablespoons (approx. 30 ml) calendula-infused olive oil
- 1 tablespoon St John's wort balsam (optional); alternatively, replace with pomegranate oil
- 2 ml (approx. 20 drops) petit grain essential oil
- 4 ml (approx. 40 drops) lavender essential oil
- 2 ml (approx. 20 drops) sweet orange essential oil
- 4 ml neroli essential oil
- 4 ml holy basil essential oil
- 2 ml lime essential oil
- 2 ml ylang ylang essential oil

*I recommend using Amphora Aromatics because, in my research, it's the best one, leaving no residue, film or grease in the bath.

Method:

1. The easiest way to do this is to pour the litre of dispersible bath oil into a large, glass measuring jug and then measure out 150 ml to keep for next time.

2. Next, add your infused oils and your avocado oil, and mix well.

3. Then, add your synergetic mix of essential oils and stir well with a glass stirring rod.

4. Finally, carefully pour your Extraordinary bath oil blend back into your litre container.

5. Enjoy!

Storage & expiry

Store in a cool, dry spot and use within six months.

Testimonial

'This bath oil is my go-to ritual when I need to unwind. The scent is calming, the texture indulgent and it leaves my skin feeling beautifully soft. It's a small luxury that I wouldn't be without!'

Lucy Jacobs

Peppermint

Peppermint has long been used for its prowess as a tummy-settler. A lesser-known use is as a tension-headache reliever, and also as a decongestant.

Latin name: *Mentha piperita*

Folk names: Mint, Brandy mint, Lamb mint

Places of origin

Believed to be a hybrid cross between watermint (*mentha aquatica*) and spearmint (*mentha spicata*), first documented in England in the late-17th century.

Description

On chocolate-brown stems, peppermint is an old familiar in the vast family of mints. Its lance-shaped leaves, with saw-toothed edges and deep-green hue, hold a vibrant oil that brightens the palate and clears the mind.

Beyond the leaf, a slender spike emerges, crowned with tiny, whorled clusters of purple or pink flowers: a subtle adornment that beckons pollinators.

Just one of over a hundred distinct varieties, peppermint releases a strong, cool, sharp aroma, spreading its squared stems and runners across the ground to form a verdant, fragrant carpet.

Historical

While other mint varieties have ancient histories, peppermint as a distinct hybrid is thought to have been first formally recognised and cultivated in England in the late-17th century. John Ray, an English naturalist, described it in 1696, and it was later formally classified by Carl Linnaeus in 1753.

Various forms of mint were used long before this, and it's likely that some ancient uses attributed to mint may have included plants that were precursors to, or early forms of, what we now know as peppermint; or simply other 'mentha' species with similar properties.

Throughout history, peppermint (or its mint relatives) has been valued for its potent aroma, refreshing taste and effectiveness in addressing digestive discomfort, and for providing a sense of clarity and invigoration. Its historical uses laid the foundation for many of the medicinal applications it's still known for today.

Mythology

In Ancient Greek mythology, Minthe was a most beautiful nymph; a loving companion to Queen Persephone, who was fated to spend the winter months of every year as queen of the Underworld.

Persephone's husband Hades became transfixed with Minthe's beauty and grace and, in usual form, badgered her to accept his ardour until she unwillingly acquiesced. On discovering their clandestine relationship, Persephone transformed Minthe into a herb: green and bushy, and rooted to the ground, with her body shrunk and withered.

Despite her new form, Minthe retained her beauty and sweetly scented aroma. Hades, saddened by the transformation, granted her the everlasting quality of aroma, whose refreshing, healing scent would persist for eternity, and whose leaves possessed universal soothing and invigorating properties – which of course, of course, mint does.

All told, there are more than 100 different varieties of mint in current cultivation, all of which smell deliciously inviting.

Medicinal uses

✓ Primarily known for its digestive benefits, helping to relieve indigestion, bloating, gas and nausea.

✓ Its antispasmodic properties can help soothe irritated bowels.

✓ Used also for headaches (especially tension headaches), muscle aches.

✓ Effective decongestant for colds and flu.

Spiritual benefits

Energising, purifying, stimulating, clarifying, uplifting.

Associated with freshness, vitality and mental clarity.

Associated chakras

Throat chakra: Associated with this chakra due to its refreshing and clarifying effect on communication and expression.

Third Eye chakra: Possesses the ability to clear the mind and enhance focus.

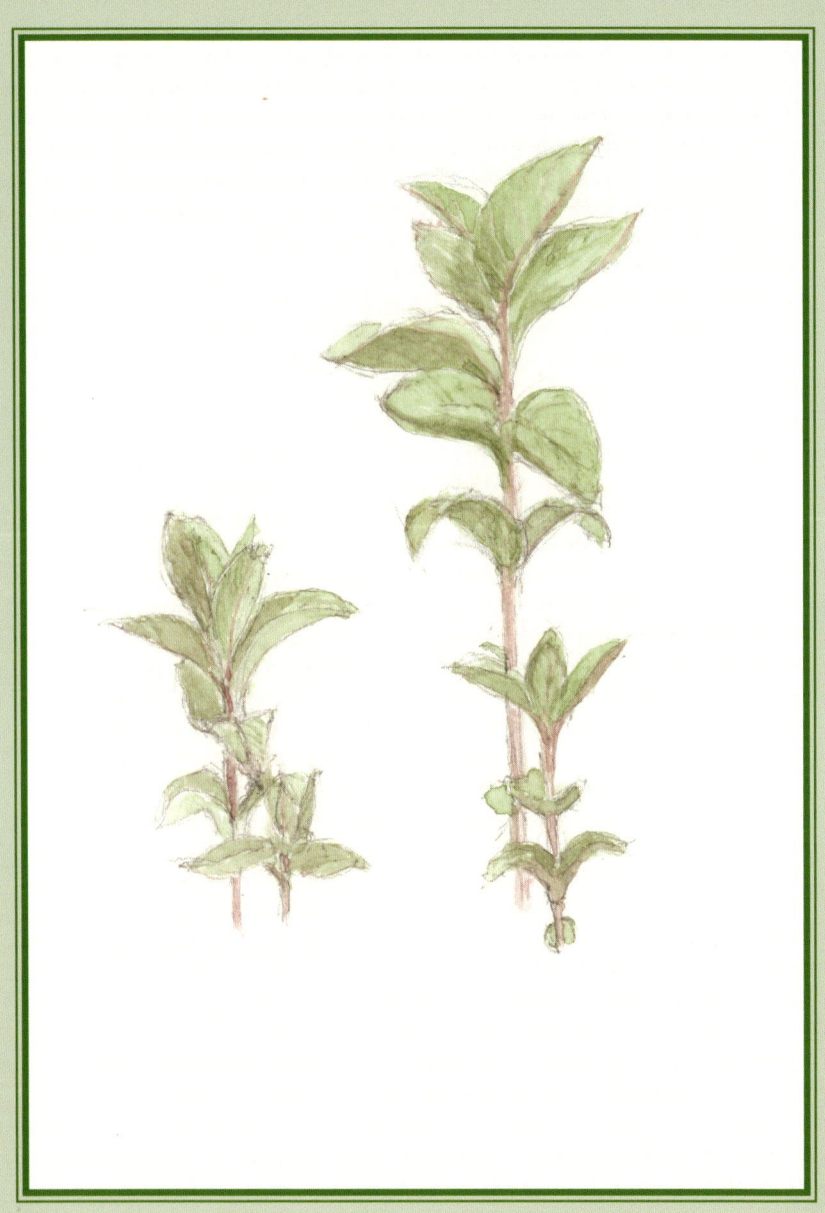

Mentha piperita

Tamara's Tales: Peppermint

I love to discover watermint in creeks and riverbanks and, in contemplative mode, watch the pink marshmallow floral puffs gently waving and rippling in the stream. I eat a lot of peppermint, too, regularly using the oil in capsules to settle my tummy, as I suffer from IBS – it helps to relax the lower intestines, reducing spasms, bloating and tummy pain.

Recipe: Minty foot balm

This balm has always been a firm favourite in my medicine chest, as it soothes, nourishes and protects sore and tired feet. It's anti-fungal, anti-bacterial, cooling, moisturising and revitalising, and helps the removal of hard skin.

The recipe below makes enough for two 100 ml jars – one for you and one for a friend!

What you'll need:

- 3 tablespoons infused oil of calendula/avocado/jojoba oil
- 1 tablespoon beeswax pellets
- 20 drops essential oil of eucalyptus
- 20 drops essential oil of peppermint
- 20 drops essential oil of lavender
- 1 tablespoon cocoa butter
- 2 tablespoons shea butter
- 50 ml witch hazel hydrosol (containing preservative)

Method:

1. Melt the plant butters, base oil and beeswax together, adding the shea butter last, when everything else is melted, to avoid it going grainy when cooled.

2. Stir well.

3. Carefully add the 60 drops of essential oil to the cooling oils and butters, and gently whisk together with a small, hand-held blender.

4. Add the witch hazel hydrosol and gently whisk to a smooth and creamy, thick emulsion.

5. Pour, spoon and scrape the whipped balm into two 100 ml, sterilised product jars and leave to cool.

6. When cool, cover with a tight-fitting lid.

7. Use after your bath or shower whenever your feet need a lift, for a lovely foot massage, or whenever your feet feel in need. (My darling daughter-in-law would have a foot massage every evening if she could!)

Storage & expiry

Store in a cool, dry place and use within six months.

Pomegranate seed oil

Pomegranate seed oil is highly prized and can be taken internally or used topically. Its benefits include skin regeneration and beautifying, and it's believed to help balance the hormones.

Latin name: *Punica granatum* (oil extracted from the seeds)

Folk names: Grenade, Apple of Granada

Places of origin

Native to the Middle East, particularly Iran and Northern India.

Description

The pomegranate contains the most beautiful, jewelled pearls, separated in pithy rills within a rubicund exterior rind. The tree is small and fiercely thorny, making collecting the fruit tricky and chance encounters with its branches quite dangerous; Nature gives not her bounty lightly where the pomegranate is concerned! Nevertheless, the fruit is used widely in Middle Eastern and Mediterranean cuisine.

Mythology

In Greek mythology, the pomegranate holds intrinsic value, used to explain seasonal change. The tale of pomegranate weaves a dance between the beautiful Persephone, daughter of Demeter and goddess of the harvest, and Hades, the all-powerful God of the Underworld.

Hades, of course, fell in unrequited love with Persephone, and enticed her to his deathly lair. There, he fed the imprisoned goddess six pomegranate seeds – signifying a contract to remain trapped with him in the depths of hell; she was bound to stay as many months as seeds she'd eaten.

Persephone's mother, distraught, allowed no flora to grow and banished all creatures from the Earth until her daughter was returned, while winter dominated, reflecting her mourning. On Persephone's return, the underworld held no sway on Earth and spring returned once more.

The tale marks a powerful reminder of the strength of a mother's love for her daughter, and her ultimate power over the very fabric of the world.

Medicinal uses

A highly prized oil, rich in punicic acid, an omega-5 fatty acid, and potent antioxidants.

- ✓ Used topically for its remarkable regenerative, anti-inflammatory and anti-aging properties for the skin. It promotes collagen production, improving skin elasticity, aiding in wound healing, and reducing the appearance of scars.
- ✓ Internally: Research suggests potential benefits for hormonal balance and heart health.

Spiritual benefits

Rejuvenating, strengthening, protective, vitalising, empowering.

Associated with fertility, abundance and renewal.

Associated chakras

Sacral chakra: For its connection to fertility, creativity and regeneration.

Root chakra: Linked with this chakra for its strengthening and grounding properties.

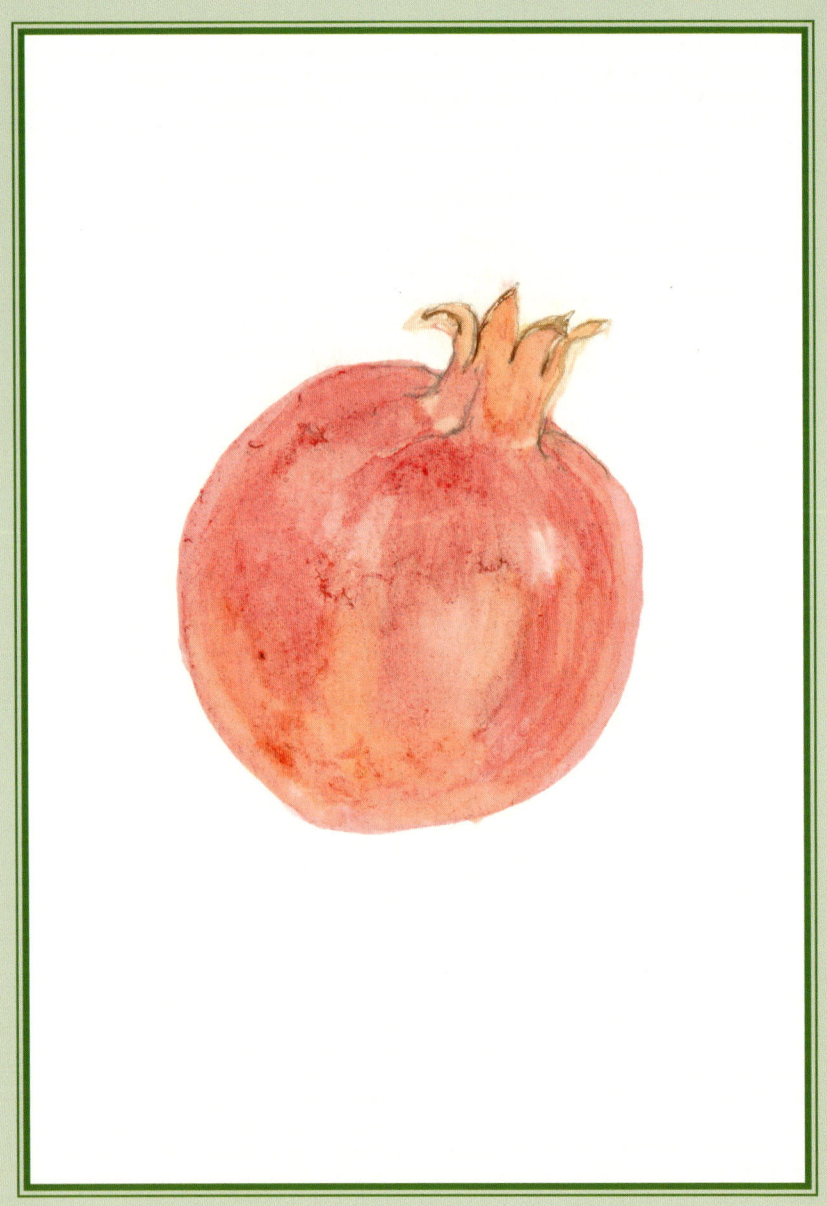

Punica granatum

Tamara's Tales: Pomegranate

Growing abundantly in Greece, I was lucky enough to have a pomegranate tree in my garden there, which fruited bountifully. The beautiful, jewelled fruit are a fabulous addition to any dish, as is the sweet extract, from which I made several tinctures and liqueurs, improving the flavour as the years went by and my skill level increased.

Pomegranate seed oil is a beautiful, deep-pink colour and smells absolutely heavenly. I was able to lay my hands on litres of it when I worked as a herbologist in the Maldives, and so experimented freely. One of my creations was a silky body butter bar for Valentine's Day, moulding it in the shape of a rose.

Recipe: Pomegranate body butter bar

My body butter bar is designed to smooth and soothe, gloss and glow, creating soft and silky, supple skin, and improving skin tone. Wonderful to ease your winter body into spring!

What you'll need:

- 6 tablespoons pomegranate seed oil
- 2 tablespoons cocoa butter
- 2 tablespoons shea butter
- 1.5 tablespoons organic beeswax
- 10 drops rose maroc essential oil
- 10 drops lavender essential oil
- 10 drops neroli essential oil
- 5 drops vanilla oil

Method:

1. Melt the oil, butters and wax together gently in a bain marie.
2. Take off the heat and allow to cool significantly – but ensure it remains as a liquid.
3. Gently stir in the synergetic essential oil mix, stirring well, until all is combined.
4. Pour into silicone moulds (I love to use rose-shaped ones for this product).

Storage and expiry

Store in a cool, dry environment. Use within two years.

Rose geranium

The oil of the rose geranium plant is used for its calming effects on the mind, while its ability to regenerate and protect the skin from damage makes it popular in skincare products.

Latin name: *Pelargonium graveolens*

Folk names: Rose-scented pelargonium, sweet-scented geranium, old-fashioned rose geranium

Places of origin

Native to the Cape Provinces and Northern Provinces of South Africa, Zimbabwe and Mozambique.

Description

The rose geranium's leaf is an intricate tapestry, deeply lobed, textured and divided, and feels like plush velvet to touch. Its flower is small and elegantly clustered, and painted in soft pink; often with two upper petals inviting a closer look, which are marked by a stroke of deeper crimson – a fleeting blush against the plant's green foliage.

When you rub its leaves between your hands, the plant releases a potent fragrance that's both sweetly floral and sharply green.

Medicinal uses

The essential oil is used in aromatherapy for its calming and uplifting properties. It's also known for its antibacterial, anti-inflammatory and astringent effects, making it useful for certain skin conditions.

✓ Used therapeutically to calm frayed nerves/reduce anxiety and stress.

✓ Anti-inflammatory: Useful in acne, eczema and minor wounds.

✓ Skin regeneration: Particularly valued in skincare for its ability to promote skin health and renewal. Its oil can assist in eliminating dead skin cells and encouraging the growth of new, healthy cells, which contributes to a more even skin tone and texture.

✓ Reduce scars and blemishes: By supporting cell regeneration, it can help diminish the appearance of scars, marks and hyperpigmentation over time.

✓ Antioxidant: Contains antioxidants that protect the skin from damage caused by free radicals and environmental stressors, which are a major factor in premature aging.

✓ Improve skin firmness: Its astringent qualities can help to tighten and tone the skin, reducing the appearance of pores and promoting a firmer, more youthful-looking complexion.

Spiritual benefits

Balancing, heart-opening, harmonising and uplifting.

Associated with love, emotional healing and self-acceptance.

Associated chakras

Heart chakra: Primarily associated with the heart centre, rose geranium is believed to help balance emotions, soothe grief and promote unconditional love.

Root chakra: Its balancing properties make it useful for grounding and connecting – a main function of the root chakra.

Tamara's Tales: Rose geranium

I first remember being fascinated with rose geranium in the Princess of Wales Conservatory at Kew gardens in London. When I discovered this plant had great therapeutic value, I was instantly hooked.

The distilled essential oil's lovely on its own and when combined with ylang ylang, lavender and neroli, in my opinion, it creates a joyful synergy for healing.

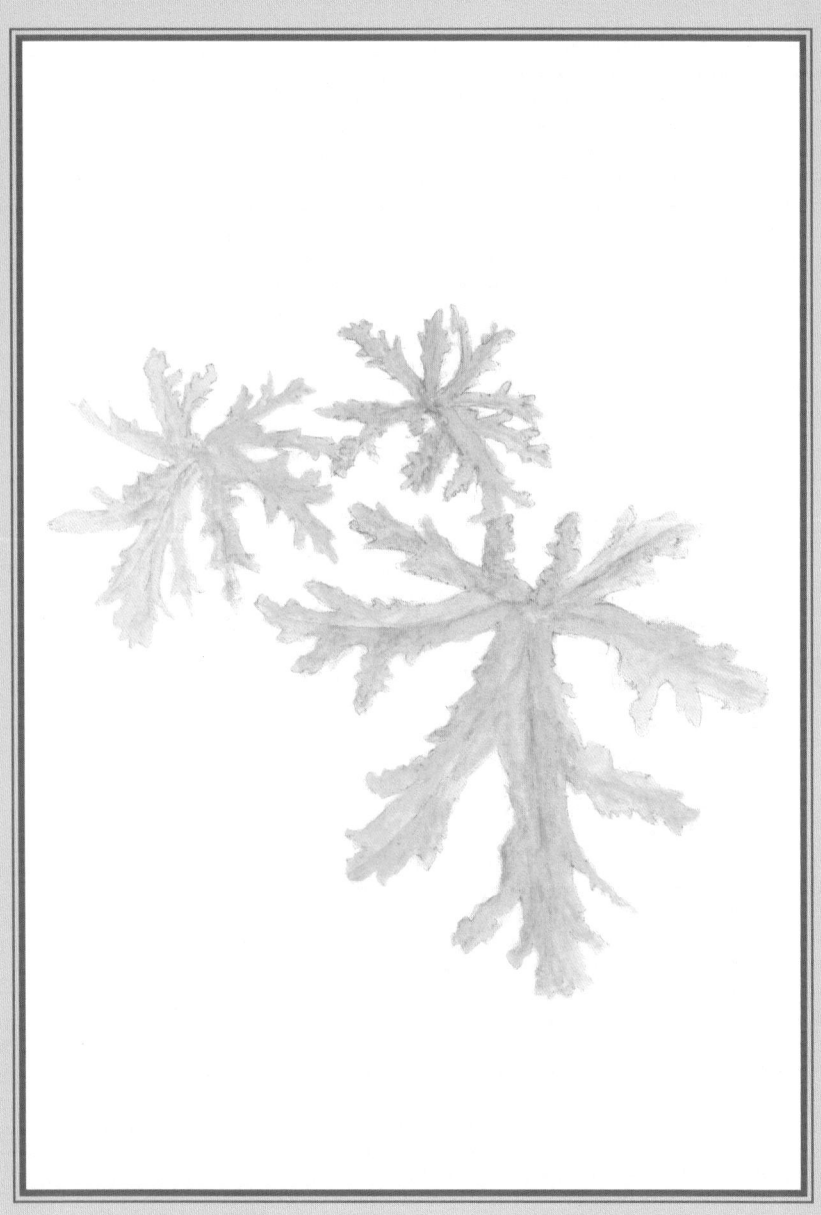

Pelargonium graveolens

To celebrate this discovery, I created a whipped body cream which I called 'Aphrodite', in homage to the incomparable Greek goddess of love, beauty, desire and pleasure, born from the foam of the sea.

Recipe: Aphrodite whipped body mousse

This gorgeous body mousse is a synergetic blend of oils combining the skin-healing properties of rose geranium with ylang ylang, lavender and St. John's wort for a super-calming, soothing and beautifully fragranced cream.

What you'll need:

- 5 tablespoons organic base face cream
- 1 tablespoon avocado oil
- 1 tablespoon calendula-infused oil
- 1 tablespoon St John's wort balsam/pomegranate oil
- 50 ml rose geranium/rose/hydrosol
- 1 ml rose geranium essential oil
- 1 ml neroli essential oil
- 1 ml ylang ylang essential oil
- 1 ml lavender essential oil
- 5 drops *immortelle/helichrysum italicum* (optional)
- 3 drops vitamin E oil
- 3 drops naturally derived preservative Benzoic acid

Method:

1. Carefully measure the base cream and plant/infused oils into a 250 ml glass measuring jug and stir together until combined.
2. Add the synergetic mix of essential oils and blend using a hand blender.
3. Then drizzle in the hydrosol, the preservative and vitamin E, and blend until fluffy and creamy.
4. Scrape or pipe into two or three sterilised, 100 ml dark glass cosmetics jars, lid and label.

Storage & expiry

Store in a cool dry spot. Use within six months.

Damask rose

Historically associated with love, the Damask rose and its essential oil are highly valued for their ability to relieve stress and open the heart. The oil is also used as a skin tonic, thanks to its anti-inflammatory properties.

Latin name: *Rosa damascena*

Folk names: Damask rose, Bulgarian rose, Taif rose, Ispahan rose, Rose of Castile

Places of origin

The precise origin of the Damask rose is debated, but it's believed to be a hybrid of *Rosa gallica* and *Rosa moschata*, originating in the Middle East. The plant has a long history of cultivation, particularly in Persia (modern-day Iran) and Bulgaria.

Essential oil derivative

Rose essential oil (Attar of Roses: a highly fragrant volatile essential oil)

Plant part: Oil extracted from fresh rose petals.

Description

The Damask rose, an empress amongst blooms, unfurls her tightly packed petals in a cascade of blush pinks and cream. Each ruffled layer holds a deep and complex fragrance: an ancient perfume, honeyed and spiced, carrying whispers of romance.

She's a flower that does not shout her beauty but harmonises with a quiet, powerful grace, her delicate head bowing gracefully on a thorny stem.

This robust, vigorous bush typically grows into a substantial shrub whose arching canes and dense, dark green foliage form a stately and fragrant presence in the garden.

Distillation: An Ancient Persian art

The extraction of the precious essence of the Damask rose is an ancient practice, perfected by the Persians centuries ago – and fascinating to explore here.

This traditional method of distillation, often involving large copper stills, allowed them to capture the volatile fragrant compounds of the rose petals, resulting in rose water and the highly concentrated essential oil known as Attar of Roses.

Freshly harvested rose petals, ideally collected in the early morning when their fragrance is most potent, were placed in the still with water. As the mixture was heated, the steam would rise, carrying the rose's aromatic molecules with it. The steam was then cooled, condensing back into a liquid. Due to the difference in density, the rose oil would separate from the rose water, allowing the precious attar, or oil, to be carefully collected.

This meticulous process, requiring vast quantities of petals for just a small amount of oil, highlights the immense value placed on the Damask rose's fragrance throughout history. A rule of thumb indicates you need about five tonnes of rose petals to produce 1kg of rose oil.

Medicinal uses

✓ Revered for uplifting the spirit and soothing emotional distress; traditionally used to alleviate stress, anxiety and depression.

✓ Aids digestion.

✓ Supports liver function.

✓ Assists in wound healing, due to anti-inflammatory and antiseptic properties.

✓ Historically, used by midwives to support childbirth.

✓ Rose water, a product of distillation, has been used as a gentle antiseptic for eyes, as well as a skin tonic.

(Aromatherapy)

Rose oil is a deeply cherished and luxurious essential oil, known for its powerful effects on emotional and mental well-being.

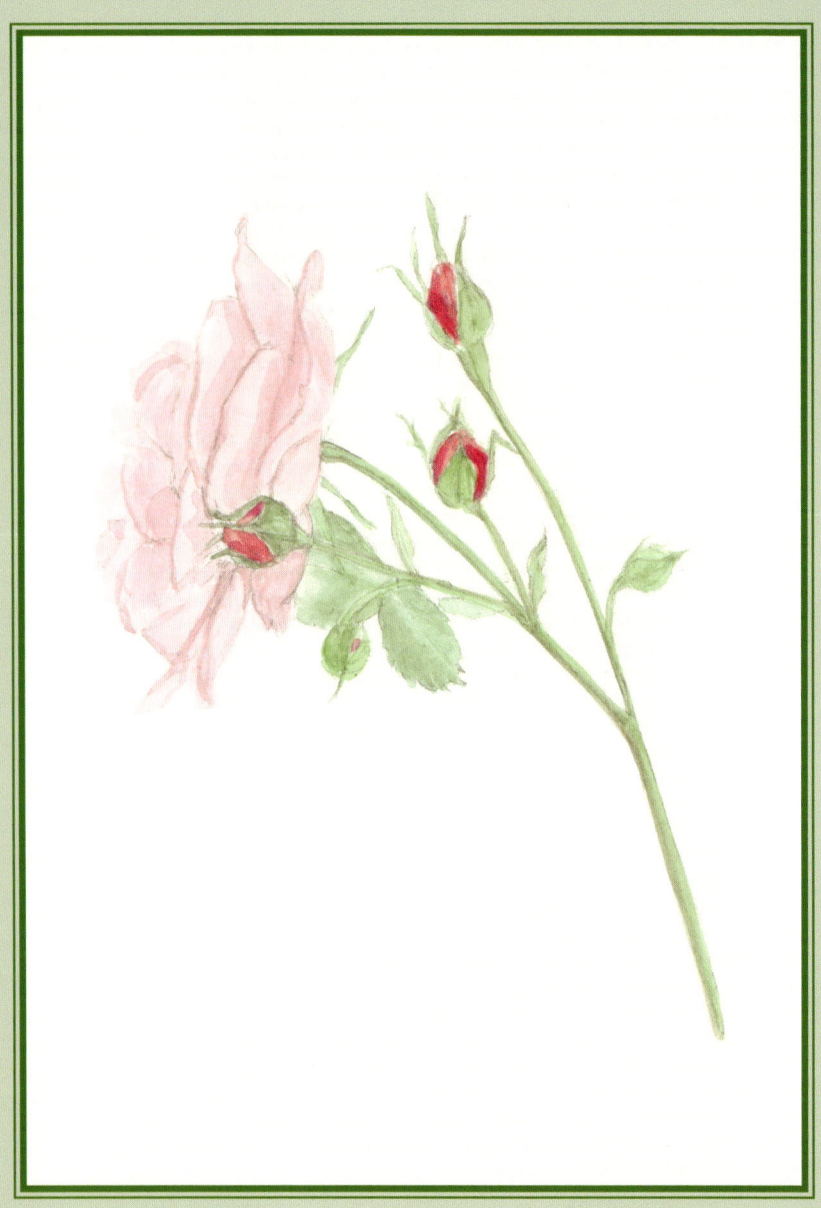

Rosa damascena

✓ Used to calm the nervous system, alleviate feelings of grief and stress, and reduce symptoms of anxiety and depression.

✓ Its exquisite floral aroma promotes feelings of love, security and happiness.

✓ Highly valued in skincare for its anti-inflammatory, astringent and regenerative properties, which help tone and rejuvenate the skin.

Spiritual benefits

Love, compassion, and emotional healing. Rose embodies a perfect balance of protective and nurturing energies, harmonising both the material and the spiritual.

Its scent is believed to open the heart and promote a sense of inner peace – elevating the soul and connecting one with a higher, more loving consciousness.

Associated chakras

Heart chakra: The Damask rose holds a powerful connection to the heart, symbolising love, compassion and emotional healing. Her traditional use in elevating mood and mitigating emotional distress resonates deeply with a balanced heart chakra.

Heart chakra: The oil is the quintessential heart-healer, helping soothe emotional wounds, open the heart to giving and receiving love, and fostering self-love and compassion.

Tamara's Tales: Damask rose

I spent several weekends in Devon, gathering material for this book with my illustrator and friend Jo. Whilst walking through her woodland and meadows, we were delighted to discover, beyond a huge bank of waist-high stinging nettles and comfrey, a beautiful Damask rose bush in full flower, which beckoned us forth and offered up the gorgeous blooms you see drawn here.

Recipe: Rose oil face mask

This beautiful evening face mask can be applied gently to the skin before a bath or bed and left to work its magic on both skin and psyche, helping you float off to sleep.

What you'll need:
- 1 tablespoon chamomile-infused oil/jojoba oil
- 50 ml Aloe vera gel
- 50 ml rose hydrosol
- 5 drops rose attar essential oil
- 5 drops lavender essential oil
- 1 drop *helichrysum italicum* essential oil (*immortelle*)
- 3 drops vitamin E oil
- 5 drops naturally derived preservative benzoic acid

Method:
1. Place the Aloe vera gel, rose hydrosol and carrier oil in a glass bowl or 250 ml glass beaker.
2. Blend together with a small, cosmetic hand blender.
3. Add the energetic essential oil mix and stir well with a glass rod.
4. Blend again with the hand blender and carefully scrape into a sterilised, 200 ml dark glass cosmetics jar.
5. Use with joy!

Storage & expiry
Store in fridge or a cool, dry, dark spot. Use within three months.

Rosemary

Rosemary is a key ingredient in any herbal collection. The oil has been shown to encourage blood flow, giving a powerful boost to the circulatory, nervous and digestive systems – perfect for soothing the tummy and increasing focus.

Latin name: *Rosmarinus officinalis* (now often classified as *Salvia rosmarinus*)

Folk names: Old Man, Dew of the Sea, Polar plant, Compass weed, Incensier

Places of origin
Native to the Mediterranean region.

Description
Rosemary has a strong heritage of culinary and cosmetic use, and is excellent as a medicinal herb due to its stimulating qualities. The plant holds a key position in aromatherapy and herbal medicine, and has long been associated in folklore with improving the memory and supporting luxuriant hair growth.

Known amongst herbalists as the 'Rose of the Mer', this association is validated by the fact that the plant inhabits well coastally. It grows vigorously both as an upright and gorgeous, creeping variety – perfect for scrambling over rocks and stones, and the purple/blue flowers are delightfully abundant.

Also known as a plant of the Sun, Rosemary is a powerful stimulant; her volatile oils have a rubifacient effect on the circulatory system, encouraging blood flow to the small capillaries of the extremities and also to the brain. For this reason, the herb can be especially useful in helping improve concentration, memory and wakefulness, while also able to reduce feelings of lethargy, dizziness and cold – which is great when caffeine isn't an option.

Medicinal uses
✓ Antioxidant and anti-inflammatory properties sometimes used to support immune health.

✓ Can stimulate circulation, relieve muscle pain and aid digestion.

✓ Traditionally used to improve memory and concentration.

Spiritual benefits
Invigorating, protective, purifying, memory enhancement, remembrance, warming.

Associated with clarity, loyalty and warding off negative energy.

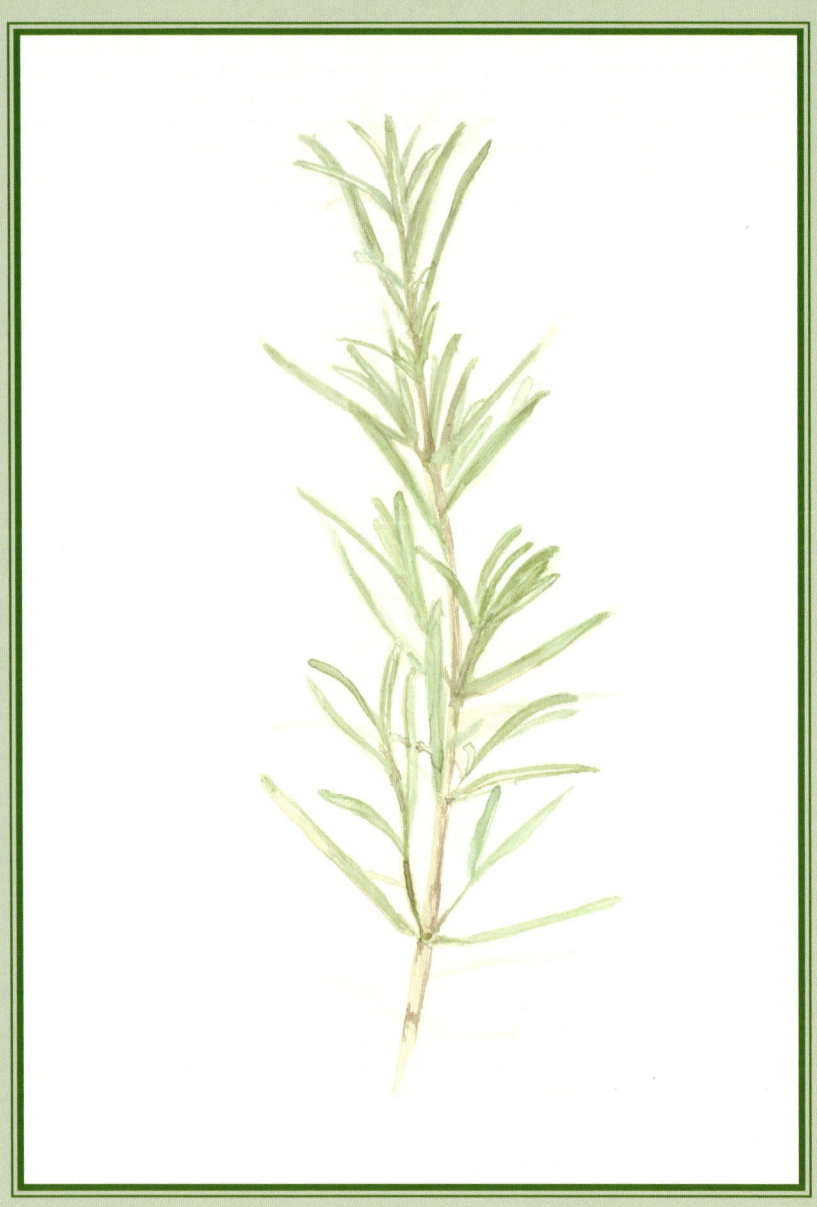

Rosmarinus officinalis

Associated chakras

Third Eye chakra: Strongly associated with the Third Eye chakra for its ability to enhance intuition, memory and mental clarity.

Solar Plexus chakra: Linked to this chakra for its warming, energising and confidence-boosting properties.

Tamara's Tales: Rosemary

To me, Rosemary's endlessly enduring, reassuringly evergreen and deeply aromatic, with a rejuvenating aroma. I've found that when held and inhaled, she offers strength and determination.

I like to combine rosemary, eucalyptus and peppermint essential oils in a synergetic blend to stay alert and focused, particularly when driving long distances.

I planted at least 80 creeping rosemary plants in the smallholding in Greece as an aromatic evergreen border plant, and grew several huge, upright bushes as hedging as well. The essential oil was easily distilled in the spring and summer, and from these wondrous drops I created the recipe below.

Recipe: Rosemary and lavender hand cream

This rejuvenating cream will protect and nurture dry winter skin, while helping to encourage circulation in the fingers to warm the hands.

What you'll need:

- 5 tablespoons organic hand cream base
- 1 tablespoon calendula infused oil
- 1 tablespoon avocado/ jojoba oil
- 5 drops vitamin E oil
- 50 ml rose hydrosol
- 2 ml (40 drops) rosemary essential oil
- 2 ml (40 drops) lavender essential oil
- 0.5 ml (10 drops) neroli essential oil
- 5 drops benzoic acid (naturally derived preservative)

Method:

1. Start by spooning the organic base cream into a 500 ml glass measuring jug.
2. Next, add the calendula and avocado oil. (If you don't have either, you can easily substitute with another lovely oil, such as pomegranate, evening primrose, jojoba or sweet almond.)
3. Add the vitamin E oil and the benzoic acid, and blend well together.
4. Then, carefully drizzle in the rose hydrosol and blend again to mix. The mixture should feel thick and creamy.
5. Finally, add the essential oils and blend again.
6. Pour or pipe the hand cream into one or two 100 ml sterilised lotion jars with a pump applicator.

Storage & expiry

Store in a cool, dry environment. Use within six months.

Ylang ylang

Known as the 'Queen of Perfumes', ylang ylang can be used to help melt away headaches, and has also gained in popularity for treating depression and for its calming effects – but this highly potent oil should be used with care!

Latin name: *Cananga odorata*

Folk names: Perfume tree, cananga, Cadmia, ilang-ilang, Fragrant cananga, macassar-oil plant, Queen of Perfumes

Places of origin

Philippines, Malaysia, Indonesia, New Guinea, Solomon Islands, Queensland, Australia, Thailand and Vietnam.

Description

The ylang-ylang flower begins its life a vibrant green. As it matures, it transforms: six long, narrow petals twist and droop gracefully as they ripen to a buttery, golden-yellow star – each petal, a slender, convoluted ribbon unfurled.

The flower itself is small but profuse, with a captivating, potent aroma wafting from the petals most strongly in the evening, ensuring the attraction of its nocturnal pollinators, moths and beetles, and enabling its intoxicating aroma to fill the tropical night.

Medicinal uses

- ✓ Widely used in aromatherapy for its calming and uplifting effects; also used for its antidepressant properties.
- ✓ Believed to relieve high blood pressure.
- ✓ Skin-supporting
- ✓ Reputedly an aphrodisiac
- ✓ Used for its antiseptic and anti-aging properties.

Spiritual benefits

Euphoric, sensual, calming, uplifting, exotic.

Associated with love, peace, joy and emotional release.

Associated chakras

Sacral chakra: Due to its connection with sensuality, creativity and emotional flow.

Heart chakra: Calming, fostering love and compassion.

Crown chakra: For spiritual connection and euphoria.

Tamara's Tales: Ylang ylang

Writing my book in Sesandan, Bali, at the edge of the Cloud Forest, surrounded by a tropical herbiary of at least 20 young ylang ylang trees, or *'Kananga'*, as they called it in Indonesia, I'm reminded of my first

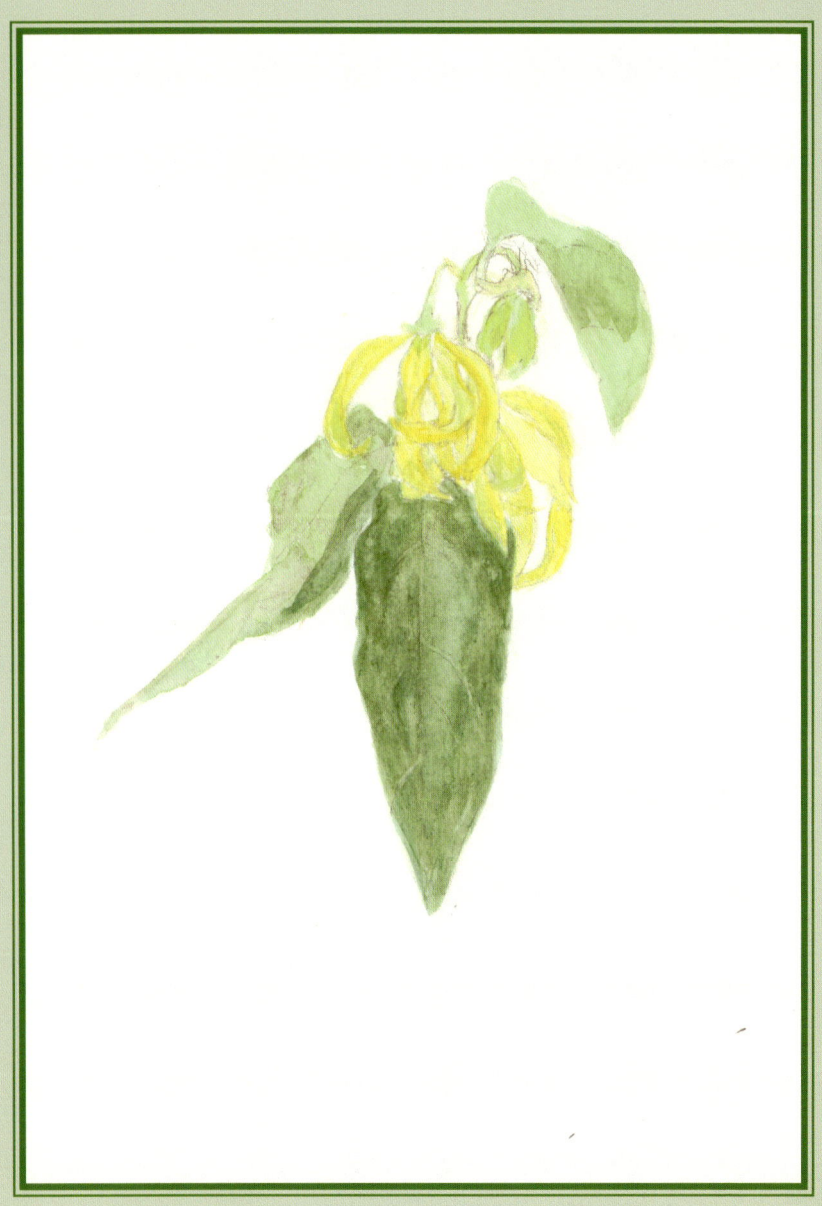

Cananga odorata

encounter with ylang ylang. It was on a family holiday in Jamaica about 30 years ago.

We were in west-central Mandeville, on a slightly hilly, cooler inland plateau, with magnificent wild horticulture such as hibiscus, mango, ackee, blue mahoe and lignum vitae, and the famous Bamboo Avenue nearby.

We were staying at a beautiful lodge, and in the centre of the courtyard was a huge ylang ylang tree, which stood at more than 100 feet high. The ground was clothed in its gorgeous flowers, whose buttery, exotic and sweet fragrance reminded me of marzipan, lemon and roses.

As we stood there, enveloped in its richness, I asked my mother what this mesmerising aroma was, and she pointed upwards towards the tree.

I was utterly intoxicated and after inhaling the ylang ylang's scent, I became suffused with a feeling I can only describe as a sense of peace and tranquillity wrapped in joyfulness!

It's a feeling I've never forgotten and it was because of that memory that ylang ylang became a staple in my aromatherapy chest.

In Bali, they use ylang ylang for skin conditions, headaches and anxiety, as a relaxant, and to treat cuts, burns and bites. They also mix it with coconut oil to make *'boori boori'* – used traditionally to protect against sun exposure and to bring down a fever.

Recipe: Rejuvenation face cream

This is the first cream I made from my Greek herbiary, using my own, distilled essential oils of lavender and rose geranium.

Ylang ylang, lavender and rose geranium combine to protect the skin, encourage skin health and cell renewal, and work with the parasympathetic system to relax and restore.

What you'll need:

- 4 tablespoons of organic base cream
- 1 tablespoon of calendula infused oil
- 1 tablespoon of chamomile infused oil

- 1 tablespoon of avocado oil
- 1 ml of lavender essential oil
- 1 ml of ylang ylang essential oil
- 1 ml of rose geranium essential oil
- 100 ml of lavender/ rose geranium/rose (your choice) hydrosol
- 1 ml of naturally derived preservative benzoic acid
- 5 drops vitamin E

Method:

1. Carefully mix the oils into the base cream in a glass bowl.
2. Add the synergetic mix of essential oils and stir well.
3. Drizzle in the hydrosol, vitamin E and preservative, and combine together with a handheld blender or small electric whisk until light and creamy.
4. Scrape or pipe into three or four clean, dark glass face cream jars.
5. Apply with joy!

Storage & expiry

Store in a cool dry spot. Use within six months.

The beautiful botanicals on the following pages don't contain a recipe, or are included in other recipes in a synergistic blend with others. Nevertheless, they're still hugely important in this collection of plant profiles.

Chamomile, for example, was an absolute must in this book because of its gentle-yet-powerful effect on the nervine system, digestion and skin health. It's included as a chamomile-infused oil in the recipe for my Calendula and chamomile skin-soothing cream, amongst others.

Similarly, avocado oil is included in many of the balms and creams in the book, and also in my 'Extraordinary bath oil' recipe. The avocado plant deserves a mention not only for its rich Caribbean heritage, but also for its huge benefits in improving the quality of our skin and hair, and its nutritional value.

Bay tree, not to be confused with *Prunus laurocerasus*, is included in the book because of its wonderful flavour and strong medicinal impact, while coconut's a staple both for cooking and its many other uses, including medicinal and therapeutic – it's absolutely wonderful as a base oil and is mentioned in many of my recipes.

Evening primrose holds a special place in my heart, supporting me when I needed it the most. With its nurturing and balancing properties, it's one of the ingredients in my calming Starflower recipe.

This book wouldn't be complete without olive oil, whose amazing benefits include skin-soothing and anti-inflammatory properties, as well as heart health when included in the diet. St. John's wort's also a treasure, and as a key plant for herbalists, is an important addition.

And finally, thyme also takes pride of place in this book. Documented in antiquity for its medicinal benefits, it's certainly worthy of a profile in the following pages. Thyme features in some of my immune-boosting recipes – pick some when you feel a cold coming on and allow it to work its magic!

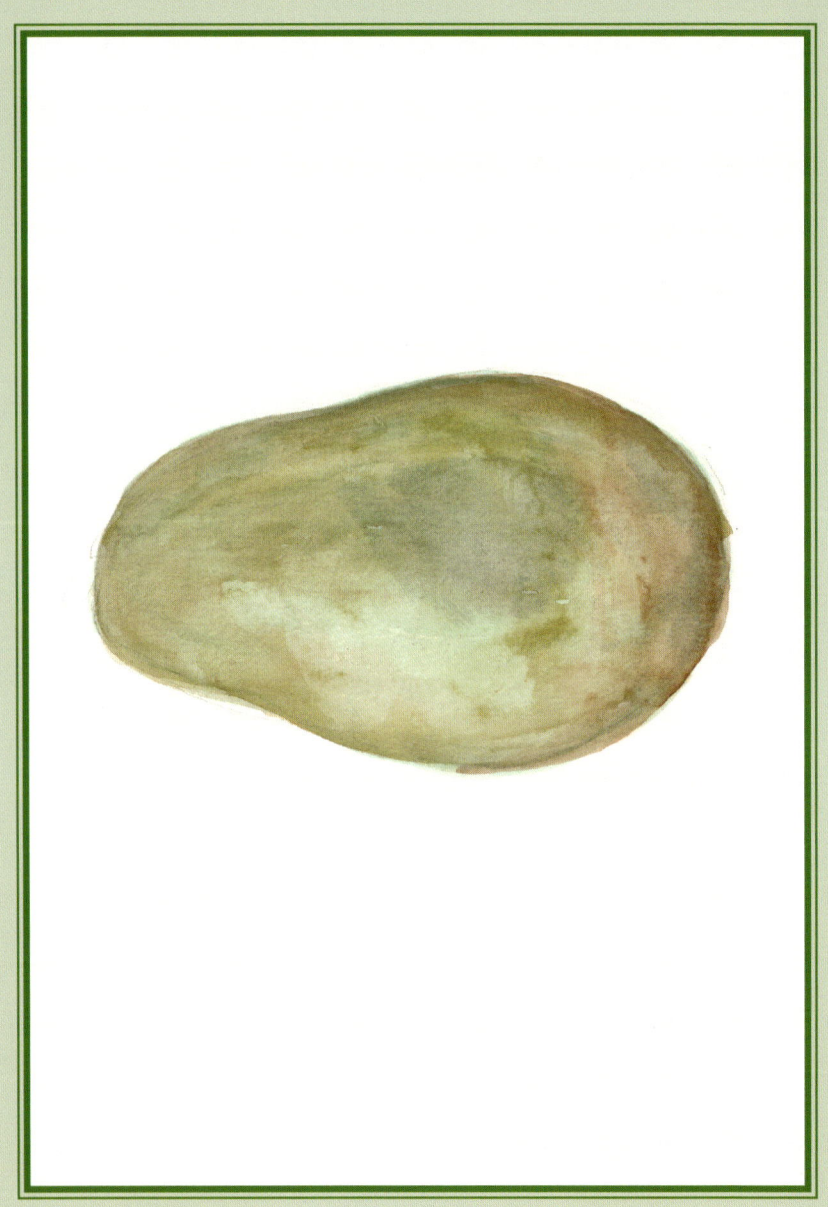

Persea americana

Avocado

Avocado is nature's powerhouse, rich in nutrients that protect the skin and support heart health.

Latin name: *Persea americana* (oil extracted from the fruit flesh)

Folk names: Alligator pear, butter fruit

Places of origin
Native to South Central Mexico.

Description
The avocado tree is a lush, sprawling evergreen that embodies a tropical richness. With its broad canopy of deep-green leaves, it offers a cool, dense shade, and its delicate, flowers of pale green or yellow give way to the promise of its singular, pear-shaped fruit.

The avocado itself, with its tough, dark skin and creamy, buttery flesh, is a symbol of nourishment and abundance, growing heavy on the branches and waiting to be picked.

The tree's quiet, steady presence in the landscape suggests a patient vitality, providing a food that's both an indulgent treat and a source of deep, healthful sustenance.

Medicinal uses
The oil of an avocado is deeply nourishing and emollient, rich in monounsaturated fatty acids, vitamins (A, D, E), and potassium. It's primarily used for:

- ✓ Moisturising, skin-softening and regenerative properties, particularly for dry, mature, or damaged skin.
- ✓ Aids in wound healing, soothes inflammation and protects against environmental damage.
- ✓ Internally: a healthy fat source, supportive of heart health.

Spiritual benefits

Nurturing, grounding, protective, enriching, supportive.

Associated with abundance, self-care and deep nourishment.

Associated chakras

Root chakra: For its grounding and nourishing qualities which support physical well-being.

Heart chakra: For promoting self-love and nurturing.

Tamara's Tales: Avocado

In the tropical islands of the Caribbean, this deep-green elixir's a cherished remedy, used not only in daily cooking but also as a traditional beauty treatment, massaged into the scalp to nourish hair and applied to the skin for a radiant, healthy glow. They simply call it 'pear' and sometimes 'butter'.

When my parents moved to Jamaica, they were lucky enough to have a huge avocado tree in their garden, which produced such quantities of fruit that a certain villager we call 'Pear Man' had grown to assume the pears were in fact his, and that he could charge a daily fee to mum and dad for the time spent picking and removing the fruits. This, he said, relieved them of the arduous task of picking and eating it.

Bay tree

The bay tree, or Laurus nobilis, is easy to grow in the garden and has long been used for a wide range of medicinal purposes, including as a digestive aid, analgesic and antiseptic.

Latin Name: *Laurus nobilis*

Folk Names: Bay, Sweet bay, Roman laurel, Poet's laurel, Daphne, Laurier

Places of origin

Native to the Mediterranean region, including Southern Europe, North Africa and Western Asia. It thrives in warm climates and well-drained soil.

Description

The bay tree is often known simply as 'bay' or 'laurel' but should *not* be confused with common Laurel (*Prunus laurocerasus*), mainly used for border hedges, which is inedible, toxic and has no medicinal properties.

Bay (*Laurus nobilis*) stands as a symbol of timeless grace and honour; its glossy, deep-green leaves holding a whisper of legend and a hint of spice.

This beautiful evergreen has smooth, grey bark and a dense, conical form. When a leaf is crushed, it releases a rich, aromatic fragrance that speaks of Mediterranean sunshine – a scent both earthy and subtly floral. The tree is a glorious plant of protection, flavour and distinction.

Mythology

Bay was held in extremely high regard by both the ancient Greeks and Romans, for whom it served as a powerful symbol of status and achievement.

In Greek mythology, bay was sacred to the god Apollo, associated with prophecy, music, poetry and healing, while its evergreen nature symbolised wisdom and immortality. Messages from Apollo were delivered by the highly influential Delphic Oracle, and the priestesses who delivered these insights reportedly chewed bay leaves to gain their prophetic visions. Additionally, the plant was central to purification rites, and was also seen as an omen for household well-being.

Meanwhile, Roman poet Ovid also immortalised the bay tree in his famed tale of Daphne and Apollo: one of love and transformation. In the fable, Apollo chided Cupid for playing with his weapons of war, whereupon Cupid shot Apollo with a magical arrow of love, causing him to develop an all-consuming desire for Daphne – and Daphne, an unmitigated loathing of Apollo.

Apollo pursued Daphne until, outrun and exhausted, she asked her father, a river god, to save her. Her father transformed his daughter into a

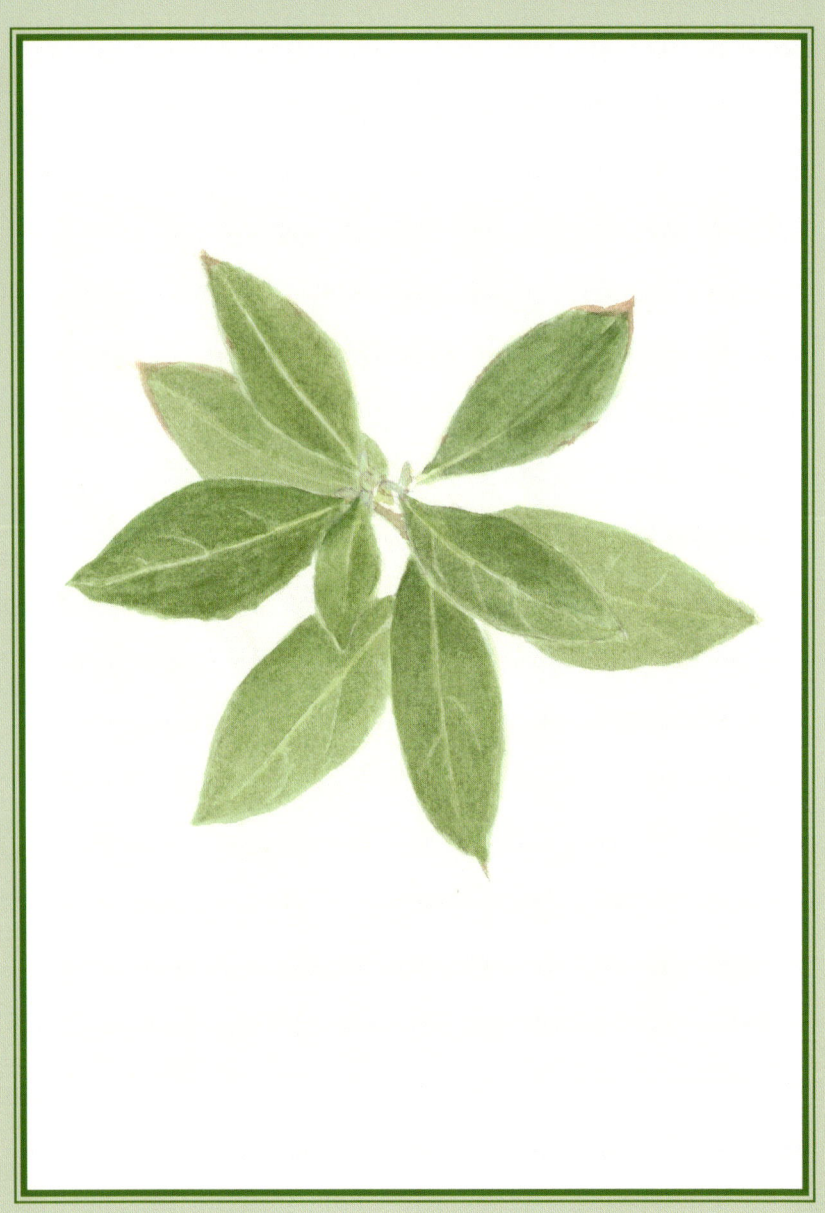

Laurus nobilis

beautiful bay tree, which stood at the water's edge. Apollo then bestowed the gift of immortality upon the laurel – hence its renown as an evergreen – and declared that her leaves would be used to make crowns for royalty, champions, victors and poets for ever after. And so, to this day, *Laurus nobilis* holds its glorious position in the forest and by streams of water.

Medicinal uses

✓ Digestive aid

Bay leaves are renowned for their carminative properties, helping to relieve indigestion, bloating and flatulence. They stimulate appetite and improve nutrient absorption. A tea made from dried leaves can soothe an upset stomach.

✓ Anti-inflammatory & analgesic

The essential oil contains compounds such as eugenol and cineole, which offer anti-inflammatory and pain-relieving effects. Topically, an infused oil or diluted essential oil can be massaged into sore muscles and joints to alleviate arthritic pain, sprains and bruises.

✓ Antiseptic & antimicrobial

Bay laurel possesses mild antiseptic qualities, making it useful in gargles for sore throats and mouth infections. Its antimicrobial action can also aid in wound healing and skin irritations when applied externally.

✓ Respiratory support

The aromatic vapours from bay leaves can help clear congested airways. Inhaling steam infused with bay leaves may provide relief from coughs, colds and bronchitis by loosening mucus and acting as an expectorant.

✓ Circulatory stimulant – traditionally used to improve circulation and promote warmth in the body.

Note on usage: While bay leaves are commonly used in cooking, medicinal applications typically involve stronger preparations like teas, tinctures, or infused oils. Always ensure proper identification and sourcing.

Consult a healthcare professional before using bay laurel medicinally, especially if pregnant, breastfeeding or on medication.

Spiritual benefits

Protective, purifying, prophetic, wisdom-enhancing. Bay is traditionally associated with victory, achievement and inspiration.

It's believed to clear negative energies and promote mental clarity.

Associated chakras

Third Eye chakra: Primarily associated with this chakra due to its connection with intuition, wisdom and prophetic vision.

Throat chakra: Resonates also with this chakra for promoting clear communication and expression.

Solar Plexus chakra: Instilling confidence and personal power.

Tamara's Tales: Bay tree

Bay's absolutely wonderful to grow in the garden, with such prolific, leafy greenery and aromatic, vigorous growth that you can give a beautiful sapling to all your friends and family within just a few years.

I put five or six large fresh bay leaves in almost every savoury dish I make – and also in my elderberry syrup and Echinacea tincture, whose recipes can be found on the elderberry and Echinacea profile pages.

Coconut

Coconut is a culinary staple. Its juices and oils are universally renowned for multiple benefits, including skin and hair nourishment, energy-boosting and antimicrobial properties.

Latin name: *Cocos nucifera*

Folk names: Tree of Life, Coco, Nariyal (Hindi), Niog (Filipino)

Places of origin

Likely Southeast Asia (specifically, the Indo-Malayan region), though widely cultivated in tropical and subtropical regions worldwide.

About

Coconut is hugely important to my botanical collection. From its husk to its shell, its leaves and oil, to its water and delicious meat, the coconut has provided communities with nourishment, shelter and even tools of civilisation for thousands of years.

Indigenous to the tropics and islands, the coconut palm is one of the most powerfully utilitarian plants known to humankind. A prolific seeder, with nuts that float across water, seeding where they wash up, the tree even inhibits coastal erosion due to its strongly rooted structure. Aptly named the 'Provision Tree' amongst the people here, it's also described as *'kalpavriksha'* – 'the All-Giving Tree' – in Indian classics, and *'pohon kelapa'* – the 'Tree of Life' – in Balinese culture.

Coconut palm holds a pivotal economic and environmental role in Tropical hemispheres, and holds a very special place in my heart. Not just a culinary staple, yielding meat, oil, water, sugar and alcohol; it's also a material resource for wood, leaves, leaf ribs, husk and shell.

The meat of the nut is a nutritious and flavourful meal, eaten both green and brown, and the oil one of the most prized and versatile in the world. Coconut water and coconut kernel contain micro minerals and nutrients essential to human health. The oil is superb for supporting the structure of the skin and hair, helping reduce scars and blemishes on the skin and adding strength, shine and gloss to the hair. People even use coconut oil to clean their teeth as well as to cook with, called 'oil pulling'.

Medicinal uses

✓ Coconut oil (from the meat) is used widely for its antimicrobial, anti-inflammatory and moisturising properties, beneficial for skin conditions and hair health.

✓ Internally: Its medium-chain triglycerides (MCTs) support energy and brain health.

✓ Coconut water is a natural electrolyte-rich rehydrator.

✓ Coconut milk is used for its nourishing properties, traditionally used for digestive issues, skin ailments and general wellness.

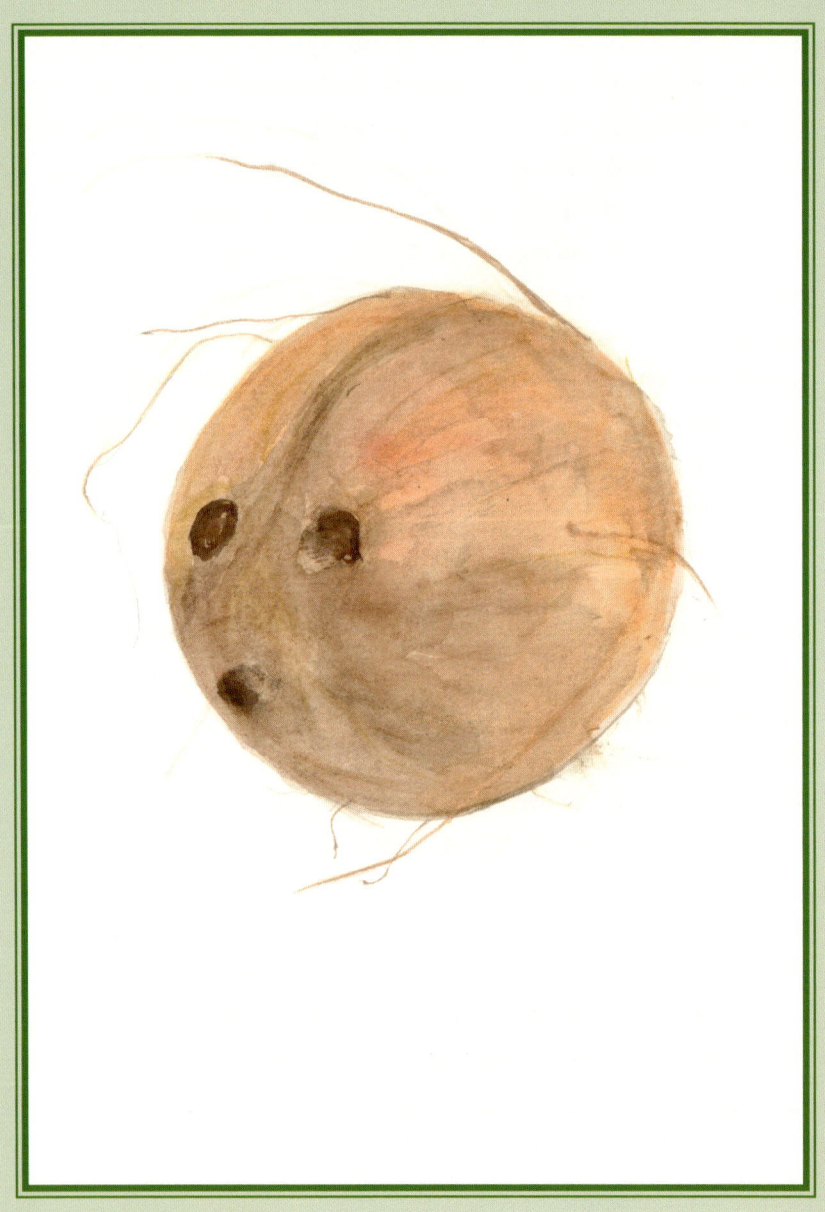

Cocos nucifera

Spiritual benefits

Nourishing, grounding, purifying, refreshing, abundant.

Associated with resilience, tropical vitality, and holistic well-being.

Associated chakras

Sacral chakra: Primarily associated with the Sacral chakra, for its nourishing and hydrating qualities, and its connection to vitality and flow.

Root chakra: For its grounding and strengthening properties, which support physical health and stability.

Tamara's Tales: Coconut

While writing this plant profile in Tarabden, Bali, I was surrounded by graceful coconut palms reaching heavenward in the gentle breeze, bursting with delicious fruit and nuts ready for picking. I was participating in a virgin coconut oil-making workshop with our Balinese hosts.

We cracked the husk and shelled the beautiful nuts before breaking apart into a bowl – five huge nuts to make our oil. We grated the glorious, flavoursome coconut meat, tasting plenty as we went, using both traditional handheld graters and more modern grating machines. The end result of our labours was an enormous pile of desiccated, sweet-smelling coconut flesh, unctuous and soft, and tasting creamy.

Then we poured the coconut water together with two pints of hot water into a bowl and squelched it together by hand, to release the precious oil from the meat. After about ten minutes of squelching and stirring, we'd separated the wonderful, milky juice from the fibrous desiccated coconut mass. There's no waste – the Balinese people use the fibres for body scrubs or animal feed.

The liquid milk containing the delicious oil was simmered for four hours to extract it the milky solids. For extra benefit, our hosts mixed in turmeric for a beautiful, buttery oil that hardens when cool. We each took a bottle home. What an amazing experience!

I love using coconut milk in my mochas, coffees and hot drinks. Any of the oils mentioned in this book and in the recipes can be replaced easily with coconut oil which, interestingly, is solid when cool but soon melts in the hand.

Chamomile

Two distinct types of chamomile can be used in aromatherapy and herbalism – although they belong to the same family, they have subtly different strengths and uses, which range from calming and soothing to anti-inflammatory.

German Chamomile *(Matricaria recutita)*

Latin name: *Matricaria chamomilla* (often seen as a synonym)

Folk names: Wild chamomile, Blue chamomile (due to the blue colour of its essential oil), scented mayweed

Roman Chamomile *(Chamaemelum nobile)*

Latin names: *Anthemis nobilis* (older, sometimes still used), *Chamaemelum nobile* (currently accepted)

Folk names: English chamomile, Garden chamomile, Low chamomile

Places of origin

- German chamomile: Native to Europe and parts of Asia, it's naturalised widely in the Mediterranean, North America and Australia. It prefers sunny locations and well-drained soil.
- Roman Chamomile: Native to Western Europe, particularly the Mediterranean region. It's commonly cultivated as a ground cover due to its low-growing habit and pleasant, apple-like scent.

Description

The chamomile plant is a gentle, low-growing herb that offers a blanket of unassuming beauty. Its delicate, finely-cut leaves create a feathery-green carpet from which thin stems rise, each crowned with a small, daisy-like flower. The blossoms, with their bright-yellow centres and pristine white petals, nod softly in the breeze, releasing a light, apple-like scent that's both calming and sweet.

This tender plant, a timeless symbol of comfort, holds its greatest power in its soothing and calming properties, which it promises in a simple cup of tea.

Medicinal uses

German chamomile is highly valued for its potent medicinal properties and is generally regarded as the stronger of the two varieties, while Roman Chamomile shares many of the same properties but's often considered milder in its action.

Their uses include:

- ✓ Anti-inflammatory: Compounds like chamazulene (which gives the essential oil its blue hue) exhibit significant anti-inflammatory effects, both internally and topically.
- ✓ Calming and sedative: Traditionally used to ease anxiety, nervousness and insomnia. It promotes relaxation and can aid restful sleep.
- ✓ Digestive aid: Helps soothe digestive upset, including bloating, gas and mild stomach cramps.
- ✓ Antispasmodic: Can help relieve muscle spasms and menstrual cramps.
- ✓ Wound healing: Topically, it can be used as a mild antiseptic and to promote the healing of minor wounds and skin irritations.

Spiritual benefits

Chamomile carries a gentle, calming and comforting energy:

Soothing and relaxing
Promotes tranquillity and helps ease emotional tension and stress.

Healing and restorative
It supports the body's natural healing processes and encourages emotional restoration.

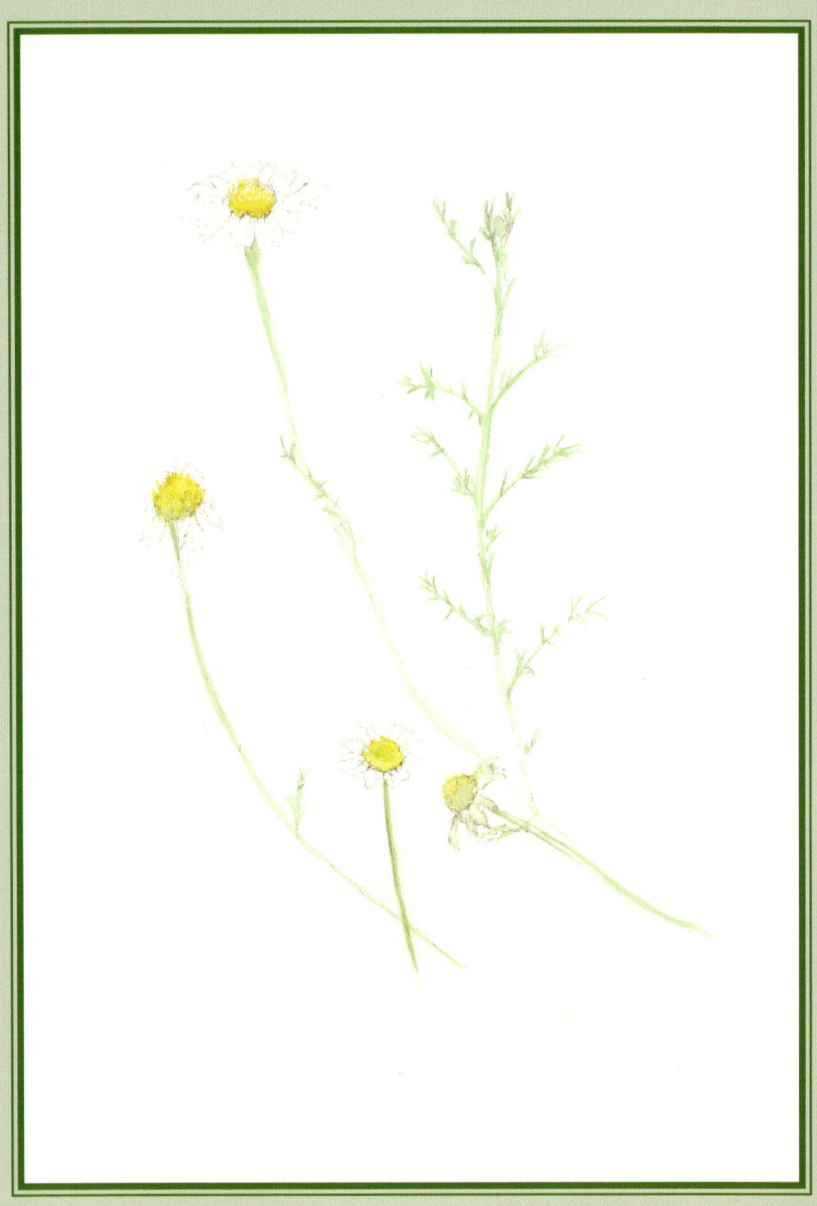

Matricaria chamomilla

Purifying
Can help to clear stagnant or negative energies, promoting a sense of lightness.

Associated chakras

Solar Plexus chakra: Because of its digestive-soothing properties and ability to ease tension.

Heart chakra: Its calming influence can also gently open and balance this chakra, fostering emotional peace and well-being.

Crown chakra: Promoting a sense of calm connection.

Tamara's Tales: Chamomile

My most potent interactions with chamomile began in Greece, when I discovered it growing in the spring along the grass ridges of the shoreline in Kalo Nero; a super-strong variety, and we made excellent tea with dried flower tops and fresh lemon balm picked from the garden as a soothing afternoon drink.

You could also buy dried packages of fabulously scented chamomile flowers, which are collected in the spring and dried in bunches over the summer, and then sold in the wonderful, local markets in the village of Kopanaki.

I tried and failed to grow chamomile in my herbal garden, but it was too dry and rocky; however, I did manage to produce a beautiful, golden-yellow infused chamomile oil using my dried chamomile flowers. I'd pack a few Kilner jars with the flowers and top off with our own locally cold-pressed virgin olive oil, and leave to infuse outside in a sunny place for a month or so. I was careful to fully cover with a layer of oil at least a centimetre above the plant materials to avoid any bacteria forming.

When the oil had taken on the sunny-yellow colour and become infused with the healing compounds, I strained it into clean oil jars for using in all sorts of lovely body butters, creams and oils. I'd also spread the plant matter into my raised planting beds to biodegrade while enriching the sandy soil.

Now, I love to use the essential oil in a synergetic blend, with lavender and neroli mixed with some calendula and chamomile-infused oil, for a beautifully soothing, deep bath before bed – sending me straight into the arms of the Greek god of dreams, Morpheus (flip over to the orange tree profile to find the recipe).

Evening primrose

Evening primrose oil is hormone-balancing, great for PMS, menopause and skin conditions – once known as the 'cure-all'.

Latin name: *Oenothera biennis*

Folk names: Evening star, Suncups, King's Cure-All, Fever plant

Places of origin
Native to North America.

Description
Evening primrose was introduced to the UK in the 1600s for medicinal and ornamental purposes, quickly establishing itself here and readily naturalising in disturbed, sandy environments due to its prolific, wind-dispersed seeds and preference for bare ground, which makes it highly adapted to dynamic habitats.

This biennial plant is surprisingly tall and resplendent, with beautiful, successive cupped lemon-yellow blooms on robust and striking stems.

While out exploring the Sea buckthorn (*Hippophae rhamnoides*) in the sand dunes at Instow, in North Devon, with this book's illustrator, Jo Thomas, we were surprised and entranced to come across a huge, naturalised community of evening primrose plants, still flowering and growing straight out of the sand. North Devon's sand dunes, such as Braunton Burrows, provide ideal conditions, thanks to their shifting sands and ongoing natural and human-induced disturbances.

Medicinal uses

- ✓ Rich in gamma-linolenic acid (GLA), the oil is widely used for hormonal balance.
- ✓ Commonly taken to alleviate symptoms of PMS, menopause and breast pain (mastalgia).
- ✓ Beneficial for skin conditions like eczema, psoriasis, and acne
- ✓ Anti-inflammatory properties also support joint health in conditions such as rheumatoid arthritis.

Spiritual benefits

Balancing, soothing, nurturing, harmonising, gentle.

Associated with emotional equilibrium, feminine wisdom and new beginnings.

Associated chakras

Sacral chakra: Primarily associated with chakra, due to its profound impact on hormonal balance and reproductive health.

Heart chakra: For its ability to soothe emotional fluctuations and promote self-acceptance.

Tamara's Tales: Evening primrose

My relationship with evening primrose oil began in my late 40s whilst recovering from an LAVH hysterectomy, due to fibroid growth. I had no idea I'd be so emotionally wrought as a consequence of losing my womb, but I was: seriously! I thought I'd lost my Root and Sacral chakras forever, and menopause hit me harder than a herd of buffalo.

I started to use the oil in combination with borage oil and *Vitex agnus casti* extract, together with clary sage essential oil and red clover extract, to try and address the emotional imbalance caused by my body not producing oestrogen anymore – at least not enough for homeostasis. This combination began to have a positive effect on my emotional state, and by degrees I felt better.

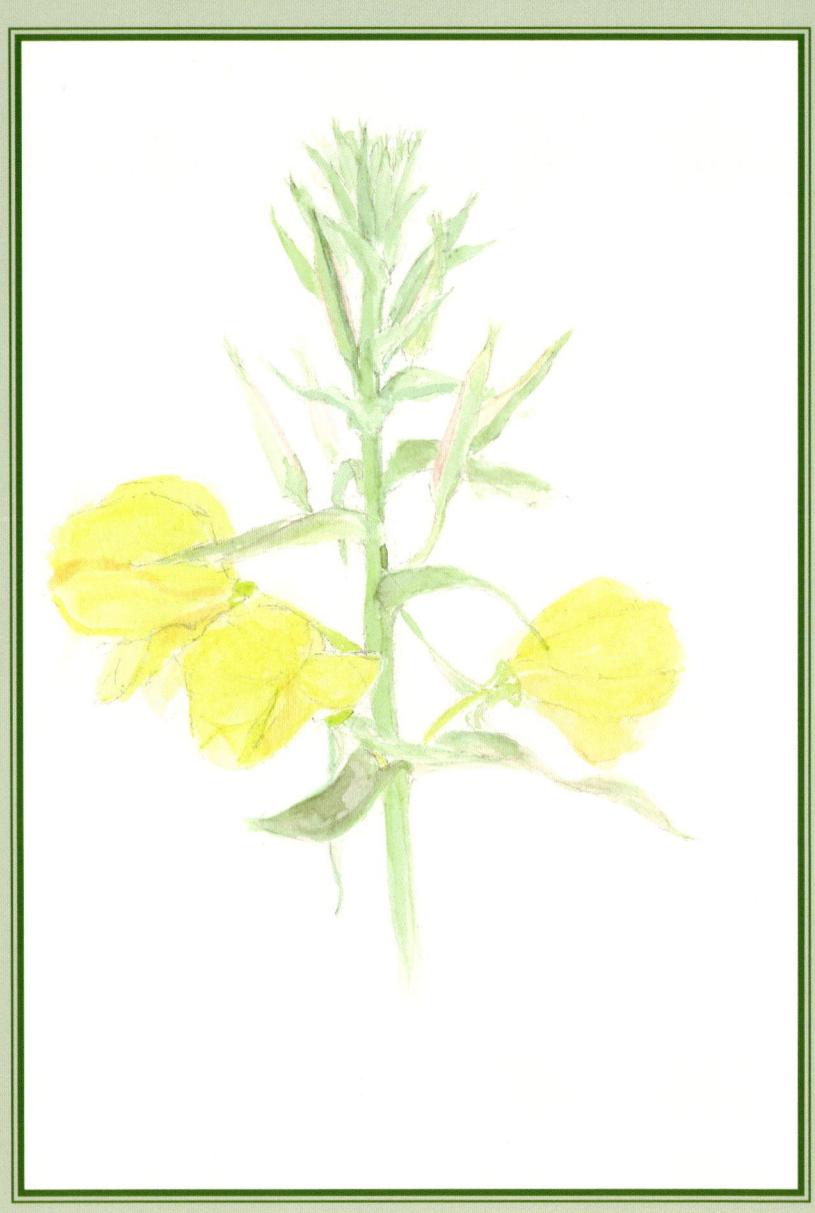

Oenothera biennis

Evening primrose has another special meaning to me: my mother has a huge specimen of it, which 'magically' appears between the paving stones on her front driveway, growing more majestically year after year, like a testament and a blessing to the feminine strength within our household.

The oil's wonderful for supporting hormonal balance, and features in my Starflower oil roller ball recipe on the borage profile page – perfect for symptoms of menopause.

Olive oil

Called 'Green Gold' for its vivid green colour as well as its significance in cooking, health benefits and as a staple part of the economy in the Mediterranean counties where it prospers.

Latin name: *Olea europaea* (oil extracted from the fruit)

Folk names: Liquid Gold, Green Gold, Oil of the Gods

Places of origin
Native to the Mediterranean Basin.

Medicinal uses
- ✓ Renowned for its heart-healthy monounsaturated fats and powerful antioxidants (polyphenols, vitamin E).
- ✓ Internally, linked to reduced risk of heart disease, stroke and certain cancers; a cornerstone of the Mediterranean diet.
- ✓ Anti-inflammatory
- ✓ Used topically: Deeply moisturising and protective for skin and hair, used for soothing dry skin, conditioning hair, and as a massage oil.

Spiritual benefits
Purifying, protective, peace-inducing, blessing, ancient wisdom.

Associated with healing, abundance and spiritual connection.

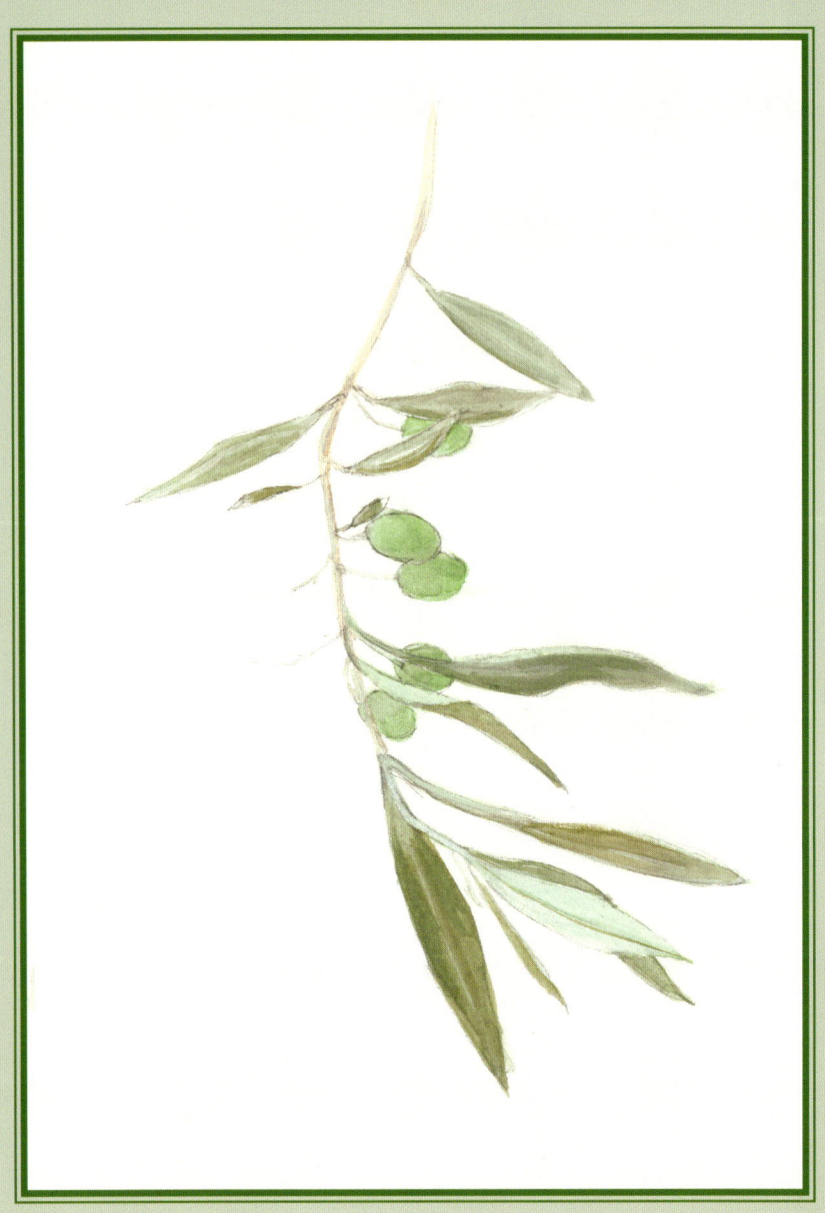

Olea europaea

Associated chakras

Heart chakra: For its profound benefits to cardiovascular health and its association with peace and compassion.

Solar Plexus chakra: Supporting overall vitality and well-being.

Tamara's Tales: The olive tree

Sitting at a taverna on the mountainside in the heart of olive-growing rural Greece, in the Southern Peloponnese region, looking out at the bay and the uninterrupted swathe of olive groves interspersed with cypress and cedar trees, I'm overwhelmed with intense gratitude and the deepest respect for Mother Nature, in all her glory. The cicadas are gently thrumming, grasshoppers and butterflies dance, and the air's balmy, while time passes unhurried and in perfect harmony with all the living things that surround.

There's an olive tree in Kalamata called the 'Mother of the Kalamata Olive', reported to be between 800 and 2,000 years old. These incredible, ancient trees stand blackened and gnarled, with silvered leaves. Their deep, thick grooves and the bonds around the trunk are a lasting testament to our healing relationship with plants and the ability of the trees to provide shelter, nutritious food, habitat, oxygen and more, to sustain the life forms around them.

I'm lucky enough to have participated in the process of organic olive oil pressing on a few occasions – from picking to pouring, and storing to sales. Olive-picking's done from late November, for the super grassy-green taste, to the end of January, which produces a smoother, more mellow flavour. At this time of year in Greece, there's a chance of huge downpours of rain, slowing everything down. There's always a sense of urgency and trepidation, as everyone rushes to get their harvest in and not mixed with anyone else's. The presses are always full to overflowing and tempers rise, as livelihoods are based on oil production.

We usually agree with our pickers to exchange goods for labour, with no actual money changing hands – the practice suits Greece's economic climate perfectly. A local Albanian family with whom we were friends would manage our harvesting – they'd gather extended family and arrive with a generator and a good few mechanical 'shakers' on poles. Thrusting the shakers high into the branches, they'd dislodge the olives into huge nets on the ground.

At the end of the pick, we'd have a lovely collection of small, lilac/black olives which would be shaken into jute sacks, to be collected by the local press four kilometres away, further down the mountainside.

We'd provide the family with plentiful food for three or four days of olive-picking from 140 or so trees, and we'd also pay for their toil with a healthy percentage of the oil produced from the harvest. The olive press would also take their tithe for the pressing and usually all parties were happy with the outcome, being well-paid in beautiful, cold-pressed extra virgin, single-estate olive oil, poured from the pressing chambers in a bright, foaming zesty green.

In addition, I was able to pick and brine several hundreds of Kalamata eating olives each year from our grove during my sojourn in Greece. The satisfaction of picking, preparing and producing fruit to table, not to mention the orange and lemon marmalade I also made, was second to none – and the taste was exquisite.

All recipes I created in Greece contained olive oil from our own olive grove; it was a privilege and an absolute joy to have had the experience of working with the wonderful 'Green Gold'.

St. John's wort

St. John's wort is a treasure used for relieving depression and uplifting the mood – however, this power-house of a plant should be used with caution, as it may interact with certain other medications.

Latin name: *Hypericum perforatum*

Folk names: St John's blood, Penny-John, Hypericum, Tipton's weed, goatweed, wound-wort, Chasse-diable

Places of origin

Native to Europe and Asia, now naturalised worldwide.

Description

St. John's wort is a cherished plant amongst herbalists. As if to herald the arrival of the summer solstice, around June in the UK, it provides a golden crown of five-petalled, vibrant star-like flowers that seem to capture the essence of the sun.

Its clustered, tiny blooms are uniquely marked with tiny, ink-black dots along their margins, with abundant feathery stamens in a central tuft. The oval leaves are so finely perforated with translucent glands that they appear pierced by countless pinpricks when held to the light: a botanical signature that inspired its scientific name.

Medicinal uses

✓ Best known for its antidepressant and mood-lifting properties, particularly for mild to moderate depression, anxiety and seasonal affective disorder (SAD).

✓ Also possesses antiviral, anti-inflammatory and wound-healing properties, used topically for burns, wounds and nerve pain, such as sciatica.

Note: Can interact with many medications.

Spiritual benefits

Brightening, protective, uplifting, strengthening, illuminating.

Associated with dispelling darkness, bringing light, and emotional resilience.

Associated chakras

Solar Plexus chakra: Strengthen personal power and alleviating emotional heaviness.

Heart chakra: For opening to joy and emotional healing.

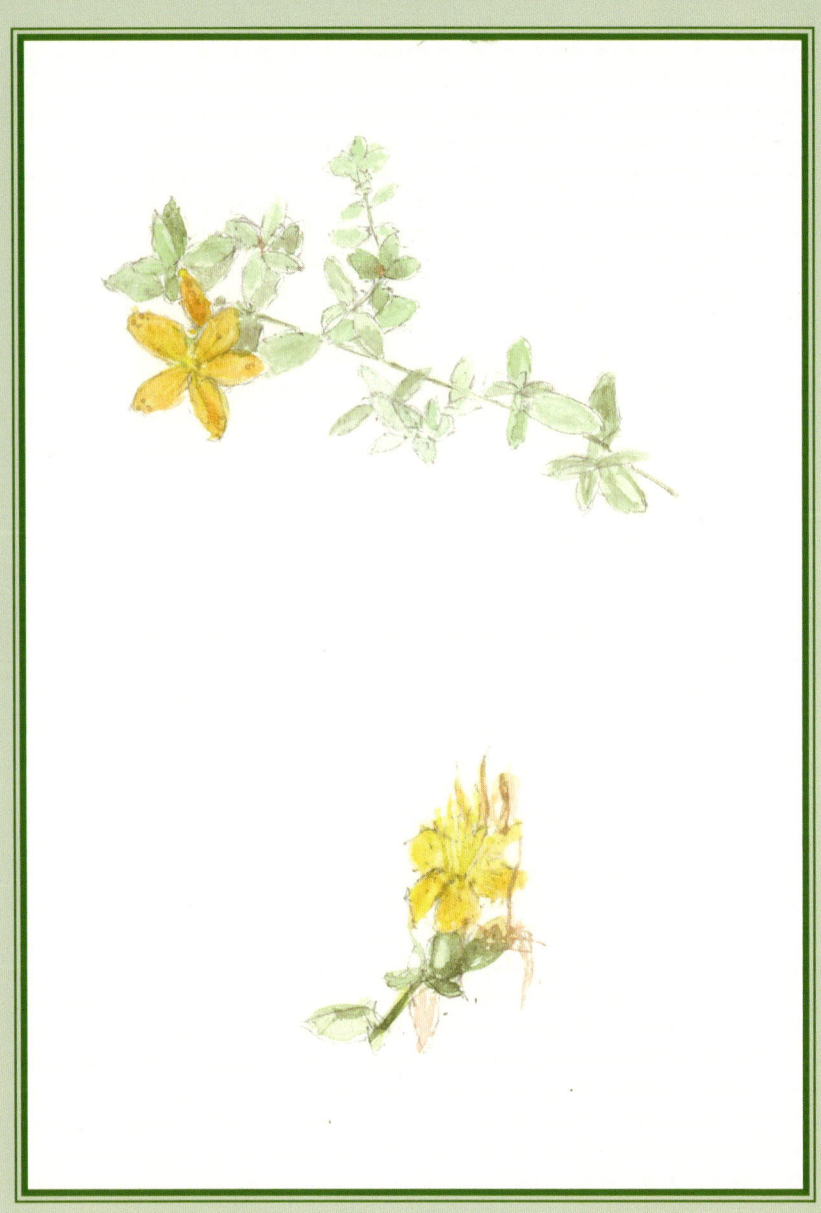

Hypericum perforatum

Tamara's Tales: St John's wort

I've included St John's wort as a comforting presence in many of my balms, creams and bath oils because I find it so soothing and uplifting – however, it's a controversial herb and cannot be used in quantities in conjunction with other medications, due to its tendency to wash them out of the body completely. In particular, it's not advised for clients taking blood thinners, blood pressure tablets or contraception, for example.

I pick the starry, flowering tops of St John's wort when I'm back in Greece, and also in the UK, and make a deep-crimson balsam for skin and hair – and just to make me feel better.

Enjoying its benefits is a simple process of wilting for a day to allow the water content to dry off (and any insects to creep away), and then steeping them in olive oil, in a warm, sunny spot in the conservatory or on the windowsill for a month or two.

When working with St John's wort, the best way to test whether the flowers are ready to pick is to crush one between your thumb and forefinger; if it leaves a maroon stain on the fingers, then it's ready to pick. Wild-harvested St John's wort, as opposed to pharmacy-bought tablets or capsules, whilst delightful to pick in the wild, though, may be of variable strength.

So, although I gladly include St John's wort in this personal selection of beautiful botanicals, if you wish to make and use your own balsam, you should consult your doctor first and research very carefully the potential interactions with any medications, as it could render the interaction unsafe.

I've therefore included an alternative oil in all cases when I've used St. John's wort balsam in my recipes in this book.

Thyme

While unassuming to look at, thyme packs a powerful punch for indigestion, and is great for treating cuts and scrapes. It's used as an ingredient in mouthwashes due to its antimicrobial properties.

Latin name: *Thymus vulgaris*

Folk names: Common thyme, Garden thyme, French thyme

Places of origin

Thyme is native to the Mediterranean region, including Southern Europe and North Africa. It's been cultivated for centuries and is now grown worldwide in various temperate climates.

Description

Thyme is a small, innocuous straggly looking herb that nevertheless packs a huge punch both aromatically and medicinally.

A staple of the herb garden, and a prolific grower in the wild on dry, stony, loamy, chalky or sandy ground, she appears in enormous variety: creeping, woolly, variegated, lemon and scented, to name a few.

Thyme provides excellent therapeutic value as a medicinal herb and as an essential oil. Her medicinal history in the British Isles is closely tied to the plant's introduction by the Romans, who used it for its aromatic and antiseptic properties. Later, herbalists like Nicholas Culpeper documented its use for respiratory ailments, headaches, and as a remedy for phlegm and shortness of breath.

The herb's highly potent antiseptic qualities were used by medics during the First World War, where her essential oil was used to sterilise hospital wards and operating theatres.

Today, the medicinal use of thyme continues, particularly in cough medicines, mouthwashes and as a traditional remedy for respiratory conditions.

Medicinal uses

Thyme is a powerful herb, primarily due to its active compounds; particularly thymol, a potent antiseptic. It's widely used for:

- ✓ Respiratory health: Thyme is a well-known remedy for coughs, bronchitis and sore throats. It acts as an expectorant, helping clear mucus from the airways, and its antimicrobial properties can help fight respiratory infections.
- ✓ Antiseptic and antimicrobial: Thyme is very effective for treating minor cuts, scrapes and skin infections when used in a diluted form. It's also used in mouthwashes and gargles to combat oral bacteria, thanks to the presence of thymol.
- ✓ Digestive aid: Thyme can help soothe tummy issues, including indigestion and gas, by promoting healthy digestion and reducing bloating.
- ✓ Antioxidant properties: Rich in antioxidants, thyme can help protect the body's cells from damage caused by free radicals.

Spiritual benefits

Thyme carries a warm, protective, and cleansing energy often associated with:

Purification and cleansing
The plant's energy is believed to clear negative vibrations from a space or from a person, making her a popular herb for smudging and energetic cleansing rituals.

Courage and strength
In ancient traditions, thyme was linked to courage and bravery. Knights would wear sprigs of the herb for protection and to bolster their courage in battle.

Emotional resilience
Thyme's energy can help fortify the spirit and provide a sense of inner strength and stability, especially during times of change or stress.141

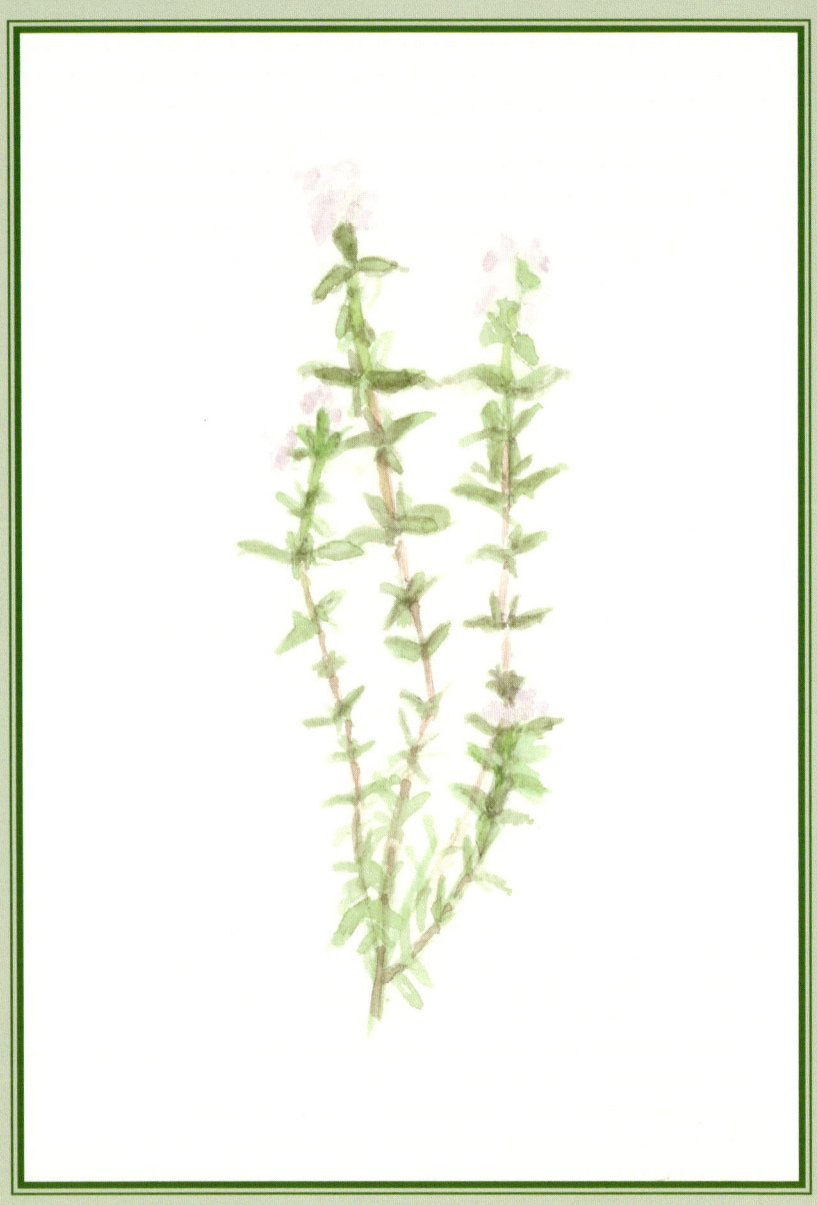

Thymus vulgaris

Associated chakras

Throat chakra: The Throat chakra governs communication and self-expression, so thyme is beneficial effects on the throat and respiratory system, combined with its energetic association with courage and speaking one's truth, align perfectly with this chakra.

Heart chakra: Its cleansing energy can also gently influence the Heart chakra, promoting emotional openness and honesty.

Tamara's Tales: Thyme

I collected some lovely wild thyme in the spring just before flowering, from a huge colony of strongly aromatic, flowering wild thyme, after coming across it on a huge hillock growing in the sand dunes whilst cycling the Kyparissia Bay, at Aianaki in Greece, and also plentifully at home in UK, in the hills and meadows of the beloved Lardon Chase, in Streatley, Berkshire – the protected home of the Chalk Hill Blue butterfly.

You'll find this wonderful herb included in my Echinacea tincture recipe to boost the immune system, and also in my Elderberry syrup, to keep flu at bay.

Reflections and Recommendations for Holistic Practice

How do holistic therapies support well-being?

Well-being is the proactive pursuit of harmonious balance across the multiple dimensions of life. The search for a calm and peaceful state of mind, with balanced energy levels and a healthy body, is the overall goal – although perceptions of physical and mental wellness, of course, are personal, individual, culturally defined and affected both by internal systems of the body and the external world around us. For all of us, however, keeping on top of well-being and self-care as a lifestyle choice is clearly a practice worth developing.

When one aspect of our well-being is unbalanced, it will often be reflected in imbalance in the other aspects. Acute stress, for example, is linked with IBS and skin conditions, and hormonal imbalances are often linked with bouts of migraine.

"It is not luxury or fine goods that produce wellbeing, but rather, a healthy balance of mind, body and soul."

Key aspects of wellness

Physical well-being

Bodily health, prevention of disease, self-care and vitality

- Skin: Often called the largest organ of the body, protecting our internal organs, regulating temperature and toxins, and release of toxins; an indicator of system health, cycles and age.
- Microbiome: Our fuel processor, navigating the processes of digestion, the problems of over-processed foods, and connecting with our psyche in the gut-brain connection.

- Systems of the body, supporting the functions of the body:
  - Circulatory
  - Respiratory
  - Lymphatic
  - Endocrine
  - Excretory

Mental well-being

Our cognitive and psychological state

- Mental health, clarity and function

- Cognitive function: emotional intelligence; resilience; mental clarity; emotional well-being; emotional regulation and self-acceptance

Social well-being

Meaningful relationships; belonging and feeling connected; contributing to the well-being of others

Spiritual well-being

Values and purpose; inner peace and harmony

Subtle energies

Understanding the concepts of Qi/Prana as a vital life force

- Meridians: Energy channels within the body

- Chakras: Perceived energy centres within the body

Environment

Connections to nature, sustainability, and safe and nurturing places

- The impact of the natural world around us; an understanding of seasonal change and how this impacts our access to plant healing.

By following the recipes in this book and learning more about botanical healing, you will decide on what works well for yourself and begin to create your own self-care pathways.

Tamara's Approach

As a lifelong educator and holistic botanical practitioner, currently working full-time in a challenging educational environment, I place a huge emphasis on physical exercise and mental relaxation in order to preserve my peace of mind and take care of my body. I love spa therapies, all types of yoga, pilates, dance and stretch exercise combined with weights and cardio in order to maintain health and fitness, as well as for mentally de-stressing.

I'm well aware of the extent to which the balance of the psyche affects all the other bodily functions. I've learnt that my energies are best focused through physical fitness and yoga early in the morning, which allows me peace of mind, body and spirit during my day. I've also learnt, through research, study and practical application, which plants and herbs support my microbiome, which essential oils support my hormones, and how to mitigate the over-production of cortisol as a physiological consequence of the unavoidable stressors of everyday life.

"If well-being is the harmonious balance of mind body and spirit, then wellness should be the positive pursuit of such a balance."

What is self-care?

Self-care represents the pathways of healing modalities alongside sensible, basic lifestyle choices: sufficient sleep, drinking enough water, participating in suitable exercise, taking time out in nature and eating nutritious food in moderation – as Hippocrates taught us more than 3,000 years ago.

This may be easy to do in theory, but in practice is not so easily achievable in our increasingly technological, always-on world. Well-being, wellness and self-care as lifestyle choices have become synonymous with a search for balance in our lives. We strive for a better work-life balance, for emotional integrity, and to juggle our household and family responsibilities with nutritional, health and fitness goals. As working individuals with or without children, we are constantly planning, organising, adapting and trying to troubleshoot several steps ahead so everything that needs to get done is done, and in good time, without mishap.

But what are the consequences of this constant race against hours in the day to achieve these complex schedules and needs? What happens to our internal balance; our need to rest and restore, to re-group our mind, body and soul? We all know the answer to that question: stress happens – the autonomic nervous system kicks in.

Understanding the parasympathetic system

The parasympathetic nervous system is one of two main branches of the autonomic nervous system (ANS), which controls our involuntary bodily functions such as heart rate, digestion and respiration. The sympathetic system primes the body for action – increasing heart rate, diverting blood to muscles, slowing digestion – while the parasympathetic system does the opposite; it acts as the body's calm-down command centre, promoting a state of relaxation and conservation of energy, and engages in restorative processes.

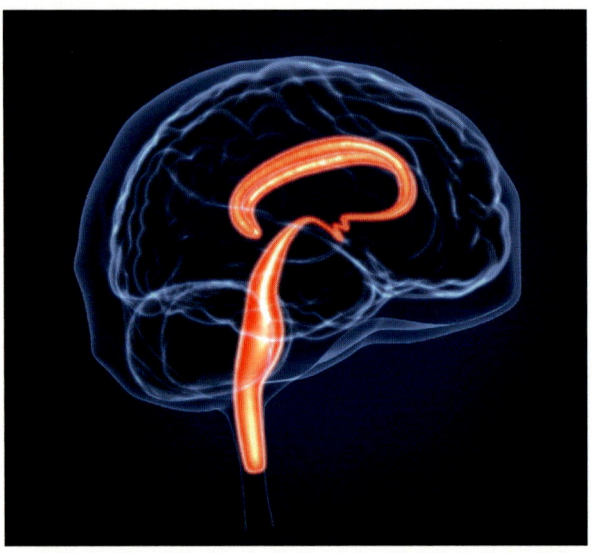

When the parasympathetic system is dominant, it signals to the body that it is safe to relax and recover; to 'rest and restore'. These signals are performed by the vagus nerve, which is the longest nerve in the autonomic nervous system. This nerve originates in the brainstem and branches out extensively, connecting to organs including the heart, lungs, digestive tract, liver and spleen.

Activation of the parasympathetic system via the vagus nerve leads to several physiological changes:

- Slowed heart rate and lowered blood pressure – reducing strain on the heart

- Improved digestion – promoting gut motility and nutrient absorption

- Relaxed muscles – releasing physical tension

- Calmed respiration – deepening and slowing breathing

- Energy conservation – shifting the body's resources towards a state of rest and restore.

Effectively, the parasympathetic system enables the body's return to its baseline state (which we can call homeostasis) after the impact of stress, supporting essential functions like digestion, detoxification, immune response and sleep.

Factors that work against the parasympathetic system

Unfortunately, many aspects of our increasingly technological lifestyle work against parasympathetic activity and keep the sympathetic system in a chronic state of low-grade activation. Persistent/chronic stress, whether from work pressure, financial worries or lifestyle, is the primary factor in the degradation of parasympathetic activity. Not enough sleep, 'grab and go' dietary choices, too little or too much exercise, constant exposure to electronic screens, and a feeling of perpetual rushing around all contribute to an imbalanced state of 'fight or flight', sympathetic dominance, and a lack of rest and restore.

Factors that support the parasympathetic system

On the other hand, activities that signal safety and relaxation to the nervous system can increase and enhance parasympathetic activity. Simple practices, such as deep, slow breathing (especially with a longer exhale); mindfulness and meditation; gentle forms of exercise such as yoga or walking in nature; laughter; sensory care, such as soothing sound baths and gentle touch; and uplifting aromas, play a significant role in shifting the nervous system towards a more relaxed state.

Botanicals, the brain and the vagus nerve

Aromatherapy and herbalism have the ability to make a significant impact on the body and mind in relieving the myriad symptoms of stress, and improving overall well-being. These practices offer potential to directly or indirectly influence the balance between the sympathetic and parasympathetic systems by acting on key pathways in the brain and body.

In order to understand how this can be possible, it is necessary to look more closely at some of the working mechanisms of the brain.

The amygdala

The amygdala is a small, almond-shaped structure located deep within the brain's limbic system. It is a super-fast emotion processor, acting as our threat detection centre; it quickly processes stimuli and, if perceived as threatening, can trigger the sympathetic, fight-or-flight response. This area of the brain also plays a large role in linking emotions to memories, designed to help us learn from past experiences by remembering what was rewarding and what was dangerous.

The reason why the amygdala, and the limbic system, play such an important role in aromatherapy is that scent has a direct pathway to the brain: the receptors in the nose send signals directly to the olfactory bulb, which is connected to the amygdala and other parts of the limbic system involved in emotion and memory. This is why an aroma can instantly evoke a memory or change our mood.

Therefore, inhalation of essential oils can directly influence the amygdala, helping reduce its alarm response. For example, the calming aromas of oils such as lavender, Melissa, neroli, chamomile, bergamot and rose interact with neurotransmitter systems in a way that promotes relaxation and reduces anxiety, helping to signal to the brain that the environment is safe. Whereas, inhaling uplifting citrus scents such as lemon, petitgrain, lime and orange can help to significantly lift the mood and spirits.

The vagus nerve

The vagus nerve, as the primary route of the parasympathetic system, offers another avenue for influence. Research suggests that some botanical compounds are able to enhance vagal tone, which is a measure of vagus nerve activity and resilience. Higher vagal tone is associated with better stress resilience and a greater capacity to move into the relaxed state.

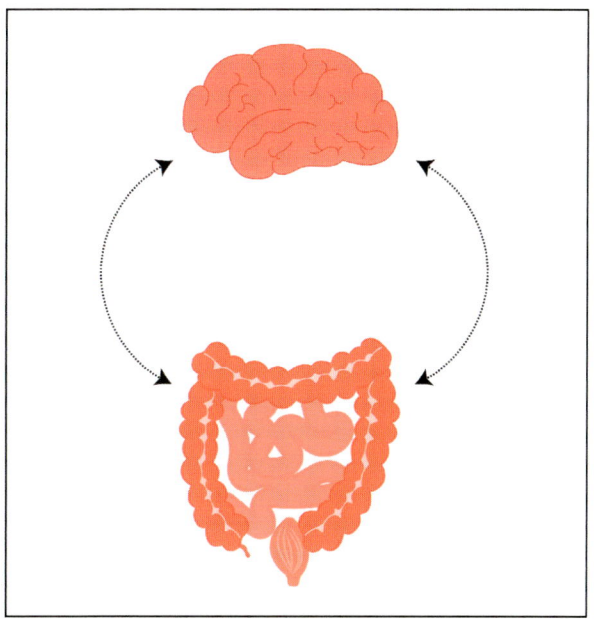

Herbal remedies can influence the ANS balance through various mechanisms, including effects that interface with the vagus nerve or reduce sympathetic drivers. For instance, calming herbal teas containing lemon balm or chamomile are traditionally used to soothe the nervous system and aid digestion; both processes that are linked to parasympathetic activity. Compounds in these herbs interact with neurotransmitter receptors or influence gut function in ways that send calming signals via the gut-brain connection, partly mediated by the vagus nerve. While the research is still developing, historical usage and contemporary experience suggest these botanicals really can help quiet the system. Topical application of essential oils in massage, for instance, combines the sensory input of aroma with the physical stimulation of touch, both known to promote parasympathetic activity and potentially influence vagal pathways.

By interacting with the amygdala and influencing vagus nerve activity, aromatherapy and herbalism offer gentle yet effective ways to help shift the autonomic balance away from fight-or-flight, sympathetic dominance and towards the rest and restore of the parasympathetic state.

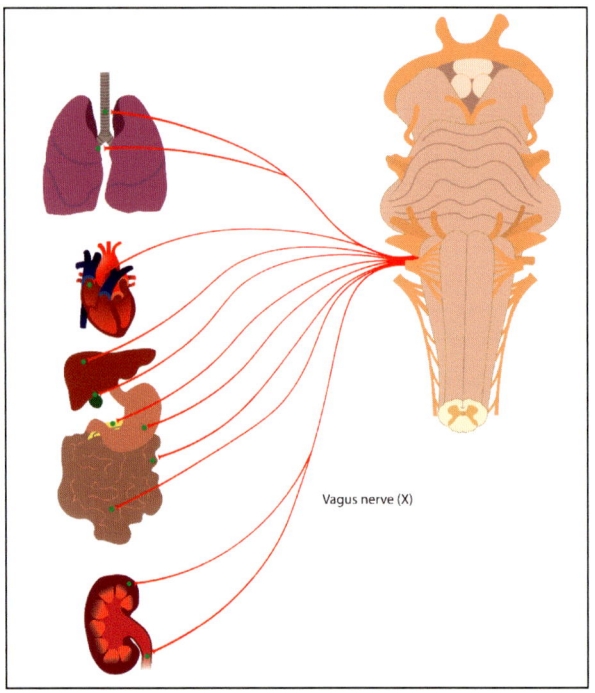

Vagus nerve (X)

Activating the rest & restore response with botanicals

Incorporating botanical healing into our daily self-care practice, then, is a really good idea. Phytotherapy can support our body's physiological responses to increase the chances of engaging a state of rest and restore, rather than having to deal with a state of alert, and then having to medicate the symptoms of stress-related illness with over-the-counter or prescription pharmaceuticals.

Botanical healing may simply involve diffusing calming essential oils into your living space regularly; choosing to take immune-boosting herbals; enjoying a warm cup of relaxing, sleep-inducing herbal tea before bed; using an essential oil rollerball blend on pulse points during stressful moments; delighting in a nightly aromatherapy bath or shower; and incorporating aromatic oils into a mindful self-massage. These practices provide sensory anchors that signal safety and calm to the nervous system, actively promoting parasympathetic activation.

Adaptogenic herbs: botanical allies in navigating stress

The formal concept of an adaptogen emerged in the mid-20th century from the research of Soviets, Dr. Nikolai Lazarev and Dr. Israel Brekhman, who tested herbs to find the best ones for helping the body resist adverse conditions without evoking the stress response. This research was driven by a desire to improve human performance and endurance, and provided a new lens through which to view and study several historically valued plants.

Based on the scientific framework that was subsequently developed, an adaptogen is a botanical agent that helps the body to cope by modulating the stress response system. Interestingly, they do not target a specific symptom but simply work to restore overall balance, or homeostasis. Unlike stimulants, which can provide a temporary boost followed by a crash, adaptogens aim to build resilience over time, helping the body cope more effectively with stress exposure without causing exhaustion or dependency.

The cultural significance of adaptogens

The use of adaptogens is deeply embedded within historical healing traditions, and while the specific term is relatively modern, the principles behind their application are ancient. Traditional systems of medicine such as Ayurveda, from India, and TCM have long recognised the value of certain plants in promoting vitality, longevity, and the ability to withstand environmental pressures. Herbs now classified as adaptogens, including ashwagandha and Holy basil (Tulsi) in Ayurveda, and ginseng and Schisandra in TCM, were traditionally employed to support the body's natural functions and help individuals maintain balance in the face of various stressors. These systems operated on a holistic understanding, viewing the body as interconnected, with resilience to challenge being paramount to health.

Adaptogenic plants

The list below includes the main, and most popular, adaptogens. Several species of fungi can also be classified as adaptogenic; however, these are not included in this list.

- Ashwagandha (*Withania somnifera*): Ashwagandha is valued for its calming properties and potential to help reduce stress and anxiety. It is often used to support adrenal function and improve the quality of sleep.

- Rhodiola (*Rhodiola rosea*): Rhodiola has been used in Scandinavian and Eastern European traditions to mitigate fatigue, enhance mental performance and improve physical endurance. It is often used for its ability to support focus and concentration.

- Ginseng (*Panax ginseng* – Asian ginseng; *Panax quinquefolius* – American ginseng): The Panax species are the most well-known adaptogens globally. Asian ginseng is traditionally used to invigorate Qi (vital energy), and to enhance physical and mental stamina. American ginseng is considered to have a milder, more cooling effect, and is often used to support the immune system and gentle stress adaptation. Both are used as tonics for overall vitality.

- Schisandra (*Schisandra chinensis*): Known in TCM for its five distinct flavours, Schisandra is used to support energy levels, improve endurance and enhance mental clarity. It is also traditionally used to support liver health and detoxification.

- Holy basil (*Ocimum sanctum/tenuiflorum*), or Tulsi: Highly revered in India, Holy basil is celebrated for its ability to help the body cope with stress, promote mental balance and support immune function. It is often consumed as a tea for its soothing effects.

- Maca (*Lepidium meyenii*): Native to the Andes mountains of Peru, maca has a long history of use by indigenous peoples for its nutritional value and its perceived ability to enhance stamina, energy and libido. It is widely used to help the body cope with stress and fatigue, and to support hormonal balance, aligning closely with adaptogenic principles.

Methods of use

Adaptogenic herbs can be incorporated into one's routine in various forms:

✓ Teas and infusions: Many adaptogens can be prepared as herbal teas, offering a simple and pleasant method of consumption, particularly for herbs like Holy basil.

✓ Tinctures: Liquid extracts in alcohol or glycerine, providing a concentrated form that is easily absorbed.

✓ Capsules and tablets: These offer a standardised dosage and are a convenient option for those who prefer not to taste the herbs directly.

✓ Powders: Ground adaptogen roots or berries can be added to smoothies, juices or other foods; an easy method to integrate them into the diet.

It is usually recommended to use adaptogens over a consistent period of time, as their effects tend to be cumulative, supporting the body's adaptive processes over time.

How do adaptogens work?

Adaptogens are thought to have an influence over the hypothalamic-pituitary-adrenal (HPA) axis. This is a network of glands and hormones located in the hypothalamus and pituitary gland in the brain, and also in the adrenal glands on top of the kidneys. Their function is to regulate stress reactions by releasing cortisol and other stress hormones from the adrenal glands. The result of this influence on the HPA axis is that adaptogens are able to help the body maintain a more balanced release of stress hormones; rather than suppressing the stress reaction, they appear to support the system in functioning more efficiently.

Studies suggest that ashwagandha may help to regulate cortisol levels, contributing to its observed effects on stress reduction and improved sleep. Rhodiola is thought to influence key stress-related pathways and neurotransmitters, potentially enhancing mental resilience and combating stress-induced fatigue. Ginseng species are believed to interact with components of the HPA axis and influence energy metabolism, supporting the body's capacity for sustained effort under stressful conditions. Maca contains compounds that may support the endocrine system, potentially contributing to its effects on energy, mood and hormonal balance in the context of stress.

Considerations and ethical practices for using adaptogens

Adaptogenic herbs can offer valuable support for well-being but, of course, must be used responsibly. Here are some key points to keep in mind:

Sustainability and ethical sourcing

As demand for adaptogens grows, especially those that are wild-harvested, concerns about over-harvesting and environmental impact increase. Choosing products that are sustainably grown or ethically sourced helps protect natural ecosystems.

Product quality and safety

The quality of herbal supplements can vary. It is best to choose brands that are transparent and perform third-party testing to confirm purity, potency and freedom from contaminants.

Possible interactions with medications

Adaptogens can interact with prescription drugs, especially those for blood pressure, blood sugar, clotting or thyroid function. If you are taking medication, consult a healthcare professional before using adaptogens.

Part of a bigger picture

These herbs work best as part of a broader healthy lifestyle. They are meant to complement – not replace – good nutrition, exercise, sleep and stress-management practices.

Stay informed

While traditional use and research are encouraging, not all claims about adaptogens are backed by strong evidence. Use credible sources and manage expectations realistically.

By approaching adaptogens with care, curiosity and respect, you can use them safely and responsibly as part of a balanced wellness routine. These herbs offer a connection to traditional plant medicine, and are validated by contemporary scientific testing into their capacity to support the body's resilience, which is why they are included in this book.

Ayurveda, TCM and a holistic view of health

Holistic practice means viewing the individual not as a collection of symptoms, but as an integrated whole. The holistic perspective considers the interconnectedness of mind, body and spirit, and, of course, is not a new invention; it has been deeply rooted in ancient healing systems developed over millennia through careful observation of nature, human physiology and the subtle interplay of life forces. The most powerful of these are Ayurveda, from India, and herbal and TCM, whose foundational principles continue to shape our understanding of holistic wellness and self-care today.

Ayurveda: the science of life

Originating in India more than 5,000 years ago, Ayurveda is often translated as the 'science of life'. Its core philosophy is that health is a state of balance and harmony between the individual's unique constitution (*prakriti*) and their environment. Ayurvedic philosophy believed that the universe, and therefore the human body, was composed of five elements – space, air, fire, water and earth – which combine to form three fundamental energies, or mind-body types, known as *doshas: vata* (air and space), *pitta* (fire and water) and *kapha* (water and earth).

Wellness through Ayurveda is achieved by keeping the doshas in balance through diet, lifestyle, daily routines, and the use of herbs and aromatic oils. Ayurveda views illness as a state of imbalance (vikriti), and seeks to restore harmony by addressing the root cause, often considering the individual's emotional and mental state alongside physical symptoms. Sensory therapies, including the use of aromatherapy and massage with oils, are integral to its approach.

Traditional Chinese Medicine & the harmony of Yin and Yang

TCM has developed over thousands of years in China, and offers another framework for understanding health and illness. Its fundamental concepts include Qi (pronounced 'chee') – often translated as 'vital energy' or 'life force' – which flows through meridians, or pathways, in the body. Health is seen as the smooth and balanced flow of Qi, along with the harmony of opposing forces known as 'Yin' and 'Yang', and the balanced interaction of the five elements of wood, fire, earth, metal and water, which correspond to different organ systems and aspects of nature.

TCM employs a variety of therapies to diagnose and treat imbalances, including acupuncture and acupressure to influence Qi flow, herbal medicine, and mindful movement practices like Qigong and Tai Chi. Like Ayurveda, TCM treats the whole person and emphasises preventing illness by maintaining balance and supporting the body's natural energetic state.

Ayurveda & TCM: shared understandings and beliefs

Despite their distinct cultural origins, Ayurveda and TCM share core principles that are important to holistic healing practice today. Both systems view the individual as an interconnected system of mind, body and spirit, inseparable from their environment. They also recognise that physical symptoms can have emotional or energetic roots, and vice versa. They both interpret internal balance as the key to wellness, rather than focusing on treating the symptoms of disease, emphasising maintaining a state of equilibrium – be it of *doshas*, Yin and Yang, the elements, or the flow of Qi.

Both approaches emphasise prevention as a cure, placing significant value on proactive self-care through appropriate diet, lifestyle and regular practices to prevent imbalances from leading to illness. Each focuses on individual treatment, recognising that each person is unique and, therefore, treatment should be personalised and based on the individual's constitution, current state of balance and specific circumstances.

Finally, they both emphasise a connection to nature, utilising plants and observing natural cycles as guides for understanding wellness and self-care therapies.

Relevance of ancient practices in modern-day healthcare

The reason these ancient principles, and the therapies they have influenced, remain so relevant today is because they offer frameworks for understanding the root causes of imbalance, and can help illustrate proactive self-care pathways – helping us meet the challenges of stress, disconnection from nature and an over-reliance on chemical pharmaceuticals for symptom management.

These practices provide guidance on diet and lifestyle, with focus on individual needs and the seasons; offer plant-based remedies for common ailments and stress support; and advocate practices like yoga, mindful movement and aromatherapy, directly countering the effects of chronic stress by promoting rest and restoring balance to the nervous system. They encourage us to develop a closer relationship with our own bodies and the natural world around us, forming a deeper connection between ourselves and our environment.

Exploring the chakras for wellness and self-care

Within the framework of the subtle energy anatomy lie key energetic junctions often referred to as 'chakras'. These are conceived as energy plug points, positioned along the central axis of the body.

Chakras are considered to be pulse points that process and distribute life force energy (Prana or Qi). Each chakra is associated with specific physical areas, emotional states, mental faculties and spiritual aspects of our being, which can influence our overall health and vitality. Understanding these energy centres offers an interesting pathway for self-awareness and holistic self-care that is echoed by, and resonates with, the botanical world.

Root chakra

Sanskrit name: Muladhara (meaning 'root support')

Colour: Red

Focus: Grounding, security, stability, survival instincts, physical identity, feeling safe in the world

Resonance
Base of the spine, pelvic floor, legs, bones, adrenal glands. It connects us to the Earth element and a sense of belonging.

How to engage:
- Participating in activities that connect you to the Earth – walking barefoot, gardening, spending time in nature
- Yoga poses like Mountain Pose, or squats
- Eating grounding foods (root vegetables)
- Practising affirmations such as, 'I am safe', 'I am grounded', 'I belong'
- Visualising red light at the base of your spine. Addressing feelings of insecurity or fear related to basic needs.

Herbal resonance
Grounding and strengthening herbs resonate here.

Use roots like ashwagandha (also an adaptogen, helping with stress-related insecurity), Valerian (for deep settling – to be used with care), or Dandelion Root (connecting to the Earth; detoxification).

Also consider using ginger and/or herbs such as rosemary and sage.

Essential oils
Black pepper, myrrh and patchouli.

Sacral chakra

Sanskrit name: Svadhisthana (meaning 'one's own abode')

Colour: Orange

Focus: Creativity, sensuality, emotions, pleasure, relationships, change, flow, passion

Resonance
Lower abdomen, sacrum, reproductive organs, kidneys, bladder. It is associated with the Water element and fluidity.

How to engage:
- Expressing creativity (e.g., art, music, dance)
- Honouring your emotions and allowing them to flow
- Engaging in activities that bring you pleasure and joy
- Connecting with water (bathing, swimming)
- Yoga poses that open the hips
- Addressing issues around control, guilt or emotional stagnation
- Affirmations like, 'I embrace pleasure', 'I am creative', 'I flow with life'
- Visualising orange light in the lower abdomen.

Herbal resonance
Herbs that support emotional flow, creativity and the reproductive system

Calendula (sunny, joyful, skin-healing – skin being a sensory organ), hibiscus (connecting to fluidity and passion); also mint, bay leaf and rose hips are useful.

Essential oils
Ylang ylang, sweet orange, rose jasmine, clary sage and cypress.

Solar Plexus chakra

Sanskrit name: Manipura (meaning 'jewel city')

Colour: Yellow

Focus: Personal power, will, self-esteem, metabolism, energy, confidence, asserting oneself

Resonance
Upper abdomen, stomach, liver, gallbladder, pancreas, diaphragm. This chakra is associated with the Fire element and transformation.

How to engage:
- Engaging in activities that build confidence (taking on challenges, setting boundaries)
- Physical exercise that strengthens the core
- Spending time in sunlight
- Practising affirmations like, 'I am powerful', 'I am confident', 'I can achieve my goals'
- Addressing issues around control, shame or low self-worth
- Visualising yellow light in the upper abdomen.

Herbal resonance:
Herbs that support digestion and metabolism, and build inner fire/confidence

Ginger (warming, digestive), peppermint (stimulating, aids digestion), lemon balm (soothes digestive upset often linked to stress; uplifting)

Rosemary can also resonate with mental clarity and confidence. Also try ginger, turmeric, chamomile and fennel.

Essential oils
Lemongrass, grapefruit, juniper and petitgrain.

Heart chakra

Sanskrit name: Anahata (meaning 'unstruck sound')

Colour: Green (primary) or pink (secondary)

Focus: Love (self-love and love for others), compassion, forgiveness, joy, connection, emotional balance

Resonance
Centre of the chest, heart, lungs, circulatory system, thymus gland. Associated with the Air element and connection.

How to engage:
- Practising compassion and forgiveness (for yourself and others)
- Spending time with loved ones
- Acts of kindness
- Connecting with nature (especially green spaces)
- Yoga poses that open the chest and shoulders
- Addressing grief, resentment or isolation
- Affirmations like: 'I am love', 'I give and receive love freely', 'my heart is open'
- Visualising green or pink light in the centre of your chest.

Herbal resonance
Herbs that support the heart (both physically and emotionally) and promote emotional opening.

Rose (a quintessential heart opener, promotes self-love), hawthorn (nourishes the physical heart, used traditionally for grief), Motherwort (calms the heart, soothes emotional stress). You can also use hibiscus, cacao and lavender.

Essential oils
Geranium, bergamot, jasmine, lavender, Melissa.

Throat chakra

Sanskrit name: Vishuddha (meaning 'especially pure')

Colour: Blue

Focus: Communication, truth, self-expression, listening, speaking your truth, creativity (expressed)

Resonance
Throat, neck, shoulders, mouth, thyroid and parathyroid glands. It is associated with the Ether/sound element, and vibration.

How to engage:
- Speaking your truth kindly but clearly

- Singing, chanting or toning

- Writing or journalling

- Active listening

- Practising conscious communication

- Addressing fear of judgment or difficulty expressing yourself

- Affirmations like, 'I speak my truth', 'I communicate clearly', 'my voice is important'

- Visualising blue light in your throat.

Herbal resonance
Herbs that soothe and support the throat, and encourage clear expression

Marshmallow root (soothing for the throat), eucalyptus or peppermint (clearing via inhalation), Red clover (traditionally associated with expression). Sage, thyme, mullein, liquorice root, slippery elm and clove are also useful here.

Essential oils
Chamomile, tea tree, frankincense and geranium.

Third Eye chakra

Sanskrit name: Ajna (meaning 'command' or 'perceive')

Colour: Indigo

Focus: Intuition, inner wisdom, imagination, clear sight, perception, psychic abilities, self-reflection

Resonance
Centre of the forehead between the eyebrows, pituitary and pineal glands, eyes, brain. Associated with Light.

How to engage:
- Meditation and mindfulness practices

- Paying attention to your intuition and dreams

- Journalling insights

- Spending time in silence

- Reducing sensory overload

- Addressing denial or resistance to inner knowing

- Affirmations like: 'I trust my intuition', 'I see clearly', 'I am connected to my inner wisdom'

- Visualising indigo light in the centre of your forehead.

Herbal resonance
Herbs traditionally used to support mental clarity, intuition and the pineal gland.

Gotu Kola (supports cognitive function; historically used for meditation), rosemary, passionflower, jasmine, Holy basil (calming, helps quiet the mind for intuition).

Essential oils
Frankincense, helicrysum, rosemary and lemon.

Crown chakra

Sanskrit name: Sahasrara (meaning 'thousand-petaled')

Colour: Violet or white/gold

Focus: Spirituality, divine connection, cosmic consciousness, enlightenment, unity, transcendence

Resonance: Crown of the head, top of the skull, cerebral cortex, pineal gland (shared with Third Eye). Associated with Consciousness itself.

How to engage:
- Meditation, prayer or contemplative practice
- Spending time in nature
- Connecting with something larger than yourself
- Practising gratitude
- Addressing feelings of separation or spiritual cynicism
- Affirmations like: 'I am connected to the Divine', 'I am one with the universe', 'consciousness flows through me'
- Visualising violet or white/gold light at the crown of your head.

Herbal resonance:
Herbs used for spiritual practice, meditation and connecting to higher states

Frankincense (traditional incense for spiritual ceremony/calming for meditation), lotus (symbolises spiritual purity and enlightenment – note that using the plant parts is less common in Western herbalism than the essence/flower), Gotu Kola (support of higher cognitive/meditative states).

Essential oils
Lavender, frankincense, sage, helicrysum, neroli, jasmine.

Working with the chakras for wellness

Working with the chakras is not about 'opening' them forcefully, but rather bringing self-awareness to these energy centres and supporting their natural, balanced flow. When our chakras are balanced, energy moves freely throughout the body, supporting physical health, emotional resilience, mental clarity and spiritual connection.

Integrating aromatherapy and herbal wellness practices provides beautiful, sensory-rich ways to connect with and support each chakra. It is a gentle, intuitive approach to self-care, acknowledging that our well-being is a dynamic interplay between the physical, emotional and energetic realms. Through an awareness of our energy centres and their interaction with botanicals, we can cultivate a deeper relationship with ourselves and enhance our capacity for wellness and self-care.

Glossary

Acupressure: A traditional Chinese medicine technique similar to acupuncture, but using physical pressure instead of needles on specific points along the body's meridians to stimulate energy flow and promote healing.

Acupuncture: A traditional Chinese medicine technique involving the insertion of thin needles into specific points on the body to stimulate energy flow (Qi) and promote healing.

Acute stress: Short-term, intense stress that can trigger the body's fight-or-flight response and, if prolonged or frequent, can contribute to various health issues.

Adaptogen: A botanical agent that helps the body adapt to stress, modulating the stress response system and promoting overall balance (homeostasis) without causing exhaustion or dependency.

Adrenal glands: Endocrine glands located above the kidneys that produce hormones, including cortisol, which are crucial for regulating metabolism, immune system, blood pressure, and the body's response to stress.

Ajna: The Sanskrit name for the Third Eye chakra, meaning 'command' or 'perceive'.

Aloe vera: A succulent plant known for its soothing and healing properties, historically used in Ancient Egyptian medicine.

Amygdala: A small, almond-shaped structure deep within the brain's limbic system, acting as a super-fast emotion processor and threat detection centre, playing a key role in the fight-or-flight response and emotional memory.

Anahata: The Sanskrit name for the Heart chakra, meaning 'unhurt' or 'un-struck'.

Ancient Egyptians: A civilisation (circa 2000 BCE) that documented the use of over 700 medicinal plants in the *Ebers Papyrus*, including Aloe vera, garlic, cannabis and frankincense.

Ancient Greece: The seat of Western civilisation from 500 BC onwards, where figures like Hippocrates and Dioscorides documented medicinal plants and promoted wellness through nutritional and herbal remedies.

Ancient Indian texts: Writings dating from 1500 BCE, such as the *Rigveda* and *Atharvaveda*, which mention the use of herbs underpinning Ayurveda.

Anti-emetic: A substance or medicine that is effective against vomiting and nausea. Many herbs, such as ginger, are known for their natural anti-emetic properties.

Aromathérapie: *Les Huiles Essentielles Hormones Végétales:* René-Maurice Gattefossé's seminal 1937 book that laid the groundwork for the modern practice of aromatherapy.

Aromatherapy: The therapeutic use of aromatic plant extracts and essential oils for psychological and physical well-being.

Ashwagandha (*Withania somnifera***):** A cornerstone adaptogenic herb in Ayurvedic medicine, valued for its calming properties, stress and anxiety reduction, and support for adrenal function and sleep quality. Also listed in ancient Indian texts.

Attar of Roses: A precious and highly concentrated essential oil extracted from the petals of various types of rose. It is a traditional perfume and medicine used in Middle Eastern and South Asian cultures, often associated with promoting emotional balance and well-being.

Atharvaveda: An ancient Indian text (circa 1500 BCE) that mentions the use of herbs underpinning Ayurveda.

Autonomic nervous system (ANS): The part of the nervous system that controls involuntary bodily functions such as heart rate, digestion, respiration and blood pressure, divided into the sympathetic and parasympathetic systems.

Ayurveda: An ancient, holistic healing system from India (more than 5,000 years old) that views health as a state of balance and harmony between an individual's unique constitution (*prakriti*) and their environment, based on the three doshas (*vata, pitta, kapha*).

Baseline state: The body's normal, resting state of physiological balance, often referred to as homeostasis.

Berries: Plant parts used as food and medicine for thousands of years.

Bergamot: An essential oil widely used for its calming and anxiety-reducing properties.

Bitumen: A black, sticky substance, historically used by the Ancient Egyptians with frankincense and myrrh for mummification, due to its preservative properties.

Black pepper: An essential oil that can resonate with the Root chakra, offering grounding and strengthening properties, and used for pain relief.

Botanicals: Plants or plant parts used for their medicinal or therapeutic properties.

Brunfels: A visionary practitioner during the Renaissance, who contributed to the development and preservation of herbal medicine.

Calendula: A herb that resonates with the Sacral chakra; known for its sunny, joyful properties and skin-healing benefits.

Cannabis: A plant listed in the *Ebers Papyrus* (circa 1550 BCE) as a medicinal plant used by the Ancient Egyptians. This plant has had a controversial medical history as, in spite of its well-documented benefits in its CBD constituent, certain strains contain dangerously psychotropic levels of THC, which makes growing and consuming the plant illegal in many countries.

Carrier oil: A vegetable-based oil (e.g., sweet almond, jojoba, coconut oil) used to dilute concentrated essential oils before topical application, to prevent irritation and ensure safe absorption.

Causae *et Curae:* A comprehensive herbal medical text produced by Hildegard of Bingen in the 12th century, detailing her considerable herbal knowledge.

Chakras: Energetic junctions or 'plug points' located along the central axis of the body, believed to process and distribute life force energy (Prana or Qi), each associated with specific physical, emotional, mental and spiritual aspects of being.

Chamomile: A calming herb traditionally used in teas to soothe the nervous system and aid digestion; its essential oil can resonate with the Solar Plexus and Throat chakras, and is used for calming and anxiety-reducing properties, and skin-soothing.

Chemical constituents: Various chemical compounds present in essential oils, each contributing to their therapeutic properties (e.g., monoterpenes, esters, aldehydes, phenols).

Clary sage: An essential oil that resonates with the Sacral and Third Eye chakras, supporting emotional flow, creativity, intuition and spiritual vision.

Cognitive function: The mental processes involved in thinking, learning, remembering, problem-solving and decision-making.

Compresses: A method of topical application where a cloth soaked in diluted essential oil is applied to the skin.

Contraindications: Specific conditions or factors that make a particular treatment or substance inadvisable.

Copper stills: Traditional distillation equipment made of copper, used to extract essential oils and hydrosols from plant material. The copper is believed to help purify the final product and improve the quality of the essential oil.

Cortisol: A primary stress hormone released by the adrenal glands, regulated by the HPA axis, which helps the body respond to stress.

Crown chakra (*Sahasrara*): The seventh chakra, located at the crown of the head, associated with spirituality, divine connection, cosmic consciousness, enlightenment, unity and transcendence; colour is violet or white/gold.

Culpeper, Nicolas: An English herbalist, physician and astrologer (1616-1654) whose works, such as *The English Physician* and *The Complete Herbal*, made herbal knowledge accessible to the public.

Cypress: An essential oil that resonates with the Sacral chakra, supporting emotional flow and creativity.

Dandelion root: A grounding herb that resonates with the Root chakra, connecting to the Earth and supporting detoxification.

Diaphoretic: A herb or substance that induces sweating, which helps to lower fever, cool the body, and promote the elimination of toxins.

Dilution: The process of mixing concentrated essential oils with a carrier oil before applying to the skin, to prevent irritation and ensure safe absorption.

Dioscorides: A figure from ancient Greece (circa 500 AD) who documented the medicinal properties of plants and promoted wellness through nutritional and herbal remedies.

Doshas: In Ayurveda, the three fundamental mind-body types or energies (*vata, pitta, kapha*), formed by the combination of the five elements, whose balance is key to health.

Ebers Papyrus: An ancient Egyptian medical text (circa 1550 BCE) that lists more than 700 medicinal plants.

Echinacea: A herb known to boost the immune system and enhance resilience to stress. It is associated with strengthening boundaries, promoting resilience and activating the body's natural defenses.

Elder tree: A plant revered in folklore as a powerful guardian. Both its flowers and berries are used medicinally, with the flowers used for respiratory issues and hay fever, and the berries used to boost the immune system and fight colds and flu.

Emotional control centre: Refers to the limbic system in the brain, which processes emotions and memory, and is directly influenced by scent.

Emotional regulation: The ability to manage and respond to an emotional experience in a way that is socially tolerable and flexible enough to permit spontaneous reactions.

Emotional well-being: A state of positive mental health whereby an individual can cope with the normal stresses of life, work productively and contribute to their community.

Empowerment: The ability of individuals to take an active role in their health care.

Endocrine: Refers to the system of glands that produce and secrete hormones directly into the bloodstream to regulate various bodily functions.

Energy conservation: The process by which the parasympathetic system shifts the body's resources towards a state of 'rest and restore', rather than expending them.

Essential oil molecules: Incredibly small molecules that allow essential oils to penetrate the skin's protective layers and enter the bloodstream.

Essential oils: Highly concentrated aromatic compounds extracted from various parts of plants, used in aromatherapy for therapeutic benefit.

Environment: The natural world around us, including connections to nature, sustainability, and safe and nurturing places, impacting access to plant healing and overall well-being.

Eucalyptus: A herb (often used as an essential oil) that can soothe and support the throat, and encourage clear expression, resonating with the Throat and Third Eye chakras. It is primarily used as a decongestant and for its clarifying and invigorating properties.

Expectorant: A substance that helps to thin and loosen mucus in the airways, making it easier to cough up phlegm. Expectorants are often used to relieve chest congestion and respiratory conditions.

Fats (lipids): Components of the skin's outermost layer (stratum corneum) which allow lipophilic essential oils to readily dissolve into and pass through.

Female healers: Women in the Middle Ages who played a fundamental role as herbalists, midwives, surgeons and traditional healers, often excluded from recorded contributions to literature and academic institutions.

Fennel: A herb that resonates with the Solar Plexus and Sacral chakras. It is known for its ability to support digestion, relieve bloating and help with hormonal balance.

Fight-or-flight: The body's natural physiological response to perceived threats, triggered by the sympathetic nervous system, preparing the body for immediate action.

Five elements (TCM): In Traditional Chinese Medicine, the five interactive phases, or energies (wood, fire, earth, metal, water), that correspond to different organ systems, emotions and aspects of nature, whose balance is crucial for health.

Frankincense: An essential oil used for meditation, calming and connecting to higher states. It resonates with the Crown, Third Eye, and Root chakras, promoting spiritual connection, mental clarity and grounding. It was also used by Ancient Egyptians for mummification, its rejuvenating effects on the skin and its anti-inflammatory properties.

Fuchs: A visionary practitioner during the Renaissance who contributed to the development and preservation of herbal medicine.

Gattefossé, René-Maurice: French chemist who coined the term 'aromatherapy' in the early 20th century, and pioneered scientific investigation into essential oils after a personal experience with lavender.

Geranium: An essential oil that resonates with the Heart and Throat chakras, promoting emotional opening and clear expression.

Gingerols: The main active compounds in fresh ginger, responsible for its distinctive flavour and many of its medicinal properties, including its anti-inflammatory and antioxidant effects.

Ginger: A warming and digestive herb that resonates with the Root and Solar Plexus chakras, supporting grounding, digestion and inner fire. Also listed in ancient Indian texts and used for pain relief.

Ginseng (*Panax ginseng, Panax quinquefolius*): Well-known adaptogens (Asian and American varieties) used to invigorate Qi, enhance physical and mental stamina, and support overall vitality and stress adaptation.

Gotu Kola: A herb that supports cognitive function and is historically used for meditation, resonating with the Third Eye and Crown chakras for higher cognitive/meditative states.

Grapefruit: An essential oil that resonates with the Solar Plexus chakra, supporting digestion and metabolism.

Gums: Plant parts used as food and medicine for thousands of years.

Heart chakra (*Anahata*): The fourth chakra, located at the centre of the chest, associated with love (self-love and love for others), compassion, forgiveness, joy and emotional balance; colour is green or pink.

Healing herbs: Plants used for their therapeutic properties to promote recovery and well-being.

Herbal apothecary: A place or practice focused on the preparation and dispensing of herbal remedies.

Herbal medicine: The practice of using plants and plant extracts for medicinal purposes.

Herbalists: Practitioners who use herbs for healing.

Herbology: The study and practice of using herbs for medicinal or therapeutic purposes.

Herbs: Plant materials that humans have used as food and medicine for thousands of years, including leaves, roots, shoots, flowers, seeds, nuts, fruits, berries, saps, gums, resins and bark.

Hildegard of Bingen: A 12th-century Benedictine nun, and one of the most famous women in the herbal tradition, who produced a comprehensive herbal medical text called *Causae et Curae*.

Hippocrates: Known as the 'Father of Medicine', from ancient Greece, he emphasised the use of herbs such as willow bark for pain relief.

Holistic medicinal solutions: Preventative and comprehensive approaches to health that consider the interconnectedness of mind, body and spirit.

Holistic perspective: A viewpoint that considers the interconnectedness of mind, body and spirit, and their inseparable relationship with the environment in understanding health and illness.

Holistic therapies: Therapeutic practices that consider the whole person – mind, body and spirit – in their approach to healing.

Holy basil (*Ocimum sanctum/tenuiflorum*), or Tulsi: A highly revered adaptogenic herb in India, celebrated for its ability to help the body cope with stress, promote mental balance and support immune function; also resonates with the Third Eye chakra.

Home remedies: Simple, traditional treatments used at home for common ailments, often involving natural ingredients.

Homeostasis: The body's ability to maintain a stable internal environment despite external changes, representing a state of physiological balance.

Hormonal imbalances: Disruptions in the body's endocrine system where hormones are either too high or too low, which can lead to various health issues.

HPA axis (hypothalamic-pituitary-adrenal axis): An intricate network of glands and hormones regulating the body's stress reaction, influencing the release of cortisol and other stress hormones.

Hydrosols: Aromatic waters produced during the distillation of essential oils, containing water-soluble plant compounds and trace amounts of essential oil.

Hypothalamus: A part of the brain that helps regulate various bodily functions, including heart rate and stress response.

IBS (Irritable Bowel Syndrome): A common disorder that affects the large intestine, causing symptoms like cramping, abdominal pain, bloating, gas and diarrhoea or constipation, often linked to stress.

Individualised treatments: Therapeutic approaches tailored to the specific needs and constitution of an individual.

Inflorescence: A cluster of flowers on a plant, arranged on a main stem. The specific shape and arrangement of the inflorescence is a key botanical characteristic, and it is a part of the plant often used in herbal medicine, such as in the case of elderflower.

Inhalation: A primary method of using essential oils in aromatherapy, where volatile aroma compounds are breathed in, directly influencing mood and the respiratory system.

Jasmine: An aromatic, floral essential oil that resonates with the Sacral, Heart and Crown chakras, supporting creativity, emotional opening and spiritual connection.

Juniper: A woody essential oil that resonates with the Solar Plexus chakra, supporting digestion and metabolism.

Jute sacks: Bags or containers made from jute, a natural plant fiber. They are often used for storing and transporting dried herbs and plant materials due to their breathability and durability.

Kapha: One of the three *doshas* in Ayurveda, representing the elements of water and earth, associated with stability, structure and lubrication.

Kilner jar: A brand of glass preserving jar with a clip-top lid and rubber seal, widely used for storing food, herbs and homemade remedies, to keep them fresh and airtight.

Lavender: An aromatic, floral multi-purpose essential oil that interacts with neurotransmitter systems to promote relaxation and reduce anxiety, resonating with the Heart and Crown chakras. Notably, René-Maurice Gattefossé observed its healing properties on a burn.

Lemon: An essential oil used to uplift mood and combat fatigue.

Lemon balm: A calming herb traditionally used to soothe the nervous system and aid digestion, often linked to stress; also uplifting, resonating with the Solar Plexus chakra.

Limbic system: A complex set of brain structures involved in emotion, motivation, memory and learning, directly influenced by scent; often called the 'emotional brain'.

Lipophilic: A property of essential oils, meaning they mix well with fats, allowing them to readily dissolve into and pass through the skin's oily barrier.

Liquorice root: A herb that can soothe and support the throat, resonating with the Throat chakra.

Lotus: A plant symbolising spiritual purity and enlightenment, whose essence/flower resonates with the Crown chakra for connecting to higher states.

Maca (*Lepidium meyenii*): An adaptogenic root native to the Andes, used for its nutritional value and perceived ability to enhance stamina, energy and libido, and support hormonal balance in the context of stress.

Malleus *Maleficarum*: A document produced in 1484 by two monks, used to justify the 'Witch Craze' during the Middle Ages.

Manipura: The Sanskrit name for the Solar Plexus chakra, meaning 'jewel city'.

Marjoram: An essential oil frequently used to promote relaxation and improve sleep quality.

Marshmallow root: A herb that soothes and supports the throat, resonating with the Throat chakra.

Massage with oils: A sensory therapy integral to Ayurveda, combining physical stimulation with aromatic oils to promote relaxation and well-being.

Marguerite, Maury: An Austrian biochemist who focused on the cosmetic and emotional applications of essential oils through massage, developing methods for their dilution and use in individualised treatments.

Meditation: A practice of focusing the mind on a particular object, thought or activity, to train attention and awareness and achieve a mentally clear, and emotionally calm, state.

Melissa: An essential oil (also known as 'lemon balm') that interacts with neurotransmitter systems to promote relaxation and reduce anxiety, resonating with the Heart chakra.

Mental well-being: Our cognitive and psychological state, encompassing mental health, clarity, function, emotional intelligence, resilience and self-acceptance.

Meridians: Energy channels or pathways in the body through which Qi (vital life force) is believed to flow in Traditional Chinese Medicine.

Microbiome: The community of micro-organisms (bacteria, fungi, viruses) that live in and on the human body, particularly in the gut, influencing digestion, immunity, and even the gut-brain connection.

Migraine: A severe headache characterised by throbbing pain or a pulsing sensation, usually on one side of the head, often accompanied by nausea, vomiting, and extreme sensitivity to light and sound; sometimes linked to hormonal imbalances.

Mindfulness: A mental state achieved by focusing one's awareness on the present moment, while calmly acknowledging and accepting one's feelings, thoughts and bodily sensations.

Monoterpenes: A group of chemical constituents found in essential oils, often in citrus and conifer oils, celebrated for their uplifting and invigorating properties.

Motherwort: A herb that calms the heart and soothes emotional stress, resonating with the Heart chakra.

Muladhara: The Sanskrit name for the Root chakra, meaning 'root support'.

Mullein: A herb that can soothe and support the throat, resonating with the Throat chakra.

Myrrh: An essential oil that can resonate with the Root chakra, offering grounding and strengthening properties. Also used by Ancient Egyptians for mummification.

Naturalised: Plants that have been introduced to an area and have established themselves in the wild.

Neanderthal man: Archaeological findings suggest prehistoric humans, including Neanderthals (dating back 60,000 years), may have used plants for medicinal purposes.

Neat (undiluted): Essential oils are rarely applied neat to the skin due to their potency, often requiring dilution in a carrier oil.

Neroli: An essential oil that interacts with neurotransmitter systems to promote relaxation and reduce anxiety, resonating with the Crown chakra.

Olfactory bulb: The brain's reception desk for smells, where signals from the olfactory epithelium are sent before heading to the limbic system.

Olfactory epithelium: A special area in the nose where tiny sensory neurons grab onto scent molecules, turning aromas into electrical signals.

Olfactory nerves: Nerves responsible for the sense of smell, providing a unique entry point for essential oils into the body.

Olfactory system: The sensory system responsible for the sense of smell, which has direct pathways to the limbic system in the brain.

Opium poppy: A plant documented by the Sumerians (3000 BCE - 500 CE) as one of the earliest recorded uses of medicinal plants.

Pain relief: A therapeutic potential of aromatherapy, where topical application of certain oils (e.g., peppermint, ginger, black pepper) may soothe muscular aches and pains.

Paracelsus: A visionary practitioner during the Renaissance who contributed to the development and preservation of herbal medicine.

Parasympathetic nervous system: One of the two main branches of the autonomic nervous system, acting as the body's calm-down command centre, promoting relaxation, energy conservation and restorative processes. Also referred to as 'rest and digest'.

Passionflower: A herb traditionally used to support mental clarity and **intuition, resonating with the Third Eye chakra.**

Patch test: A safety measure performed before applying a new essential oil liberally to the skin, to check for individual sensitivity.

Patchouli: An essential oil that can resonate with the Root chakra, offering grounding and strengthening properties.

Peppermint: A stimulating and digestive herb (often used as an essential oil) that aids digestion and can be clearing via inhalation, resonating with the Solar Plexus and Throat chakras. Also used to uplift mood, combat fatigue, and for respiratory support and pain relief.

Pharmacology: The branch of medicine concerned with the uses, effects and modes of action of drugs.

Phytotherapy: The use of plants for medicinal purposes; plant healing.

Pitta: One of the three doshas in Ayurveda, representing the elements of Fire and Water, associated with metabolism, transformation and heat.

Plant healing: The therapeutic use of plants for health and well-being.

Plant oils and extracts: Concentrated forms of plant compounds, often used in herbal medicine and aromatherapy.

Prana: In Ayurvedic philosophy, universal life energy or vital life force, often associated with breath.

Prakriti: In Ayurvedic philosophy, an individual's unique constitution or inherent nature, determined at conception.

Preventative health care: Focuses on preventing illness and maintaining long-term wellness.

Qi: In Traditional Chinese Medicine, vital life force or energy that flows through meridians in the body; also a concept of vital life force in general.

Qigong: A traditional Chinese mind-body practice that involves slow, deliberate movements, deep breathing and meditation to cultivate and balance Qi.

Renaissance: A period of significant development and preservation in the field of herbal medicine, bringing a revival of classical texts and new contributions.

Resins: Plant parts used as food and medicine for thousands of years.

Respiratory support: A therapeutic potential of aromatherapy, where certain essential oils are used via inhalation to help clear congestion and support respiratory function.

Rest and digest: A state promoted by the parasympathetic nervous system, focusing on relaxation, energy conservation and restorative bodily processes.

Rhizome: A horizontal, underground plant stem that can produce new roots and shoots. Many medicinal plants, such as ginger and turmeric, have rhizomes that are used for their therapeutic properties.

Rhodiola (Rhodiola rosea): An adaptogenic herb found in cold, high-altitude regions, used to combat fatigue, enhance mental performance and improve physical endurance, especially under duress.

Rigveda: An ancient Indian text (circa 1500 BCE) that mentions the use of herbs underpinning Ayurveda.

Rose: A quintessential heart-opening herb and essential oil that promotes self-love and emotional opening, resonating with the Heart and Sacral chakras.

Rose hips: A herb that resonates with the Sacral chakra, connecting to fluidity and passion.

Rosemary: A herb and essential oil that can resonate with the Root, Solar Plexus, and Third Eye chakras, supporting grounding, mental clarity, confidence and intuition.

Sacral chakra (*Svadhisthana*): The second chakra, located in the lower abdomen, associated with creativity, sensuality, emotions, pleasure, relationships and flow; associated colour is orange.

Safe absorption: The process by which essential oils are absorbed into the body without causing harm, typically ensured by proper dilution.

Sage: A herb and essential oil that can resonate with the Root, Throat, and Crown chakras, offering grounding, soothing and spiritual properties.

Sahasrara: The Sanskrit name for the Crown chakra, meaning 'thousand-petaled'.

Schisandra (Schisandra chinensis): An adaptogenic herb known in TCM for its five distinct flavours, used to support energy levels, improve endurance, enhance mental clarity and support liver health.

Scientific inquiry: A new age of investigation spurred by technological advancements during the Industrial Revolution, casting doubt on traditional herbal practices.

Self-care: The proactive pursuit of practices and lifestyle choices that support one's physical, emotional, mental and spiritual well-being.

Seven chakras: The seven main energy centres located along the central axis of the body, from the base of the spine to the crown of the head.

Shen Nong Ben Cao Jing: The earliest Chinese medical text (circa 2800 BCE), attributing knowledge of 365 medicinal plants to the mythical Emperor Shen Nong.

Side-effects: Unintended and often undesirable effects of medications. Herbal remedies generally have a lower incidence of these compared to pharmaceuticals.

Skin: The largest organ of the body, protecting organs, regulating temperature, releasing toxins and indicating overall system health.

Skin care: A therapeutic potential of aromatherapy, where diluted essential oils are used to support skin health.

Slippery elm: A herb that can soothe and support the throat, resonating with the Throat chakra.

Solar Plexus chakra (*Manipura*): The third chakra, located in the upper abdomen, associated with personal power, will, self-esteem, metabolism, energy and confidence; associated colour is yellow.

Spiritual well-being: A sense of purpose, meaning and connection to something greater than oneself, often involving inner peace and harmony.

Steam inhalation: An active method of inhalation where essential oils are added to hot water, and the steam is inhaled.

Stratum corneum: The outermost protective layer of the skin, through which essential oil molecules can slip.

Stress reduction and mood enhancement: A therapeutic potential of aromatherapy, where many essential oils are used for their calming, anxiety-reducing, uplifting and fatigue-combating properties.

Stress reaction: The body's physiological and psychological response to stressors, mediated by the HPA axis and the autonomic nervous system.

Subtle energies: Concepts like Qi, Prana, the meridians and chakras, which describe vital life forces and energy channels within the body.

Sumerians: A civilisation (3000 BCE - 500 CE) that left some of the earliest recorded uses of medicinal plants on clay tablets.

Svadhisthana: The Sanskrit name for the Sacral chakra, meaning 'one's own abode'.

Synergistic essential oil blend: A combination of two or more essential oils where their combined therapeutic effect is strengthened and more powerful than the sum of their individual parts.

Symbiotic relationship: A close and long-term interaction between two different biological organisms, as seen between humans and the plant kingdom.

Sympathetic system: One of the two main branches of the autonomic nervous system, which primes the body for action, increasing heart rate, diverting blood to muscles, and slowing digestion ('fight-or-flight').

Synthetic drugs: Lab-made medicines created by isolating active compounds from plants, which can be standardised, accurately dosed and mass-produced.

Systems of the body: Major physiological systems, including the circulatory, respiratory, lymphatic, endocrine and excretory systems, that support bodily functions.

Tai Chi: A traditional Chinese martial art and mind-body practice involving slow, flowing movements, deep breathing and meditation for health and well-being.

Taoist: Pertaining to Taoism, a Chinese philosophical system that emphasises living in harmony with the Tao (the natural order of the universe).

Tea tree: An essential oil that can soothe and support the throat, resonating with the Throat chakra. Also used for respiratory support and blemishes.

Therapeutic potential: The capacity of a substance or practice to produce beneficial healing effects.

Theophrastus: An apprentice of Hippocrates from ancient Greece, who helped document the medicinal properties of plants.

Third Eye chakra (*Ajna*): The sixth chakra, located at the centre of the forehead, associated with intuition, inner wisdom, imagination, clear sight and self-reflection; its associated colour is indigo.

Throat chakra (*Vishuddha*): The fifth chakra, located in the throat, associated with communication, truth, self-expression and listening; associated colour is blue.

Thyme: A plant documented by the Sumerians (3000 BCE - 500 CE) as one of the earliest recorded uses of medicinal plants. Also, a herb that can soothe and support the throat, resonating with the Throat chakra.

Tinctures: Liquid extracts of herbs, providing a concentrated form that is easily absorbed and convenient for precise dosing.

Topical application: A primary method of using essential oils in aromatherapy whereby diluted oils are applied to the skin for local and systemic effects.

Toxicity: The degree to which a substance can harm an organism – a concern with internal consumption of essential oils.

Traditional Chinese Medicine (TCM): An ancient, holistic healing system from China that views health as the smooth and balanced flow of Qi, harmony of yin and yang, and balanced interaction of the Five elements.

Turmeric: A herb that resonates with the Solar Plexus chakra, supporting digestion and metabolism. Also listed in ancient Indian texts.

Valmet, Jean: A French physician who used essential oils to treat injured soldiers during the Second World War, documenting their therapeutic effects.

Vagal tone: A measure of vagus nerve activity and resilience; higher vagal tone is associated with better stress resilience and a greater capacity to move into a relaxed state.

Vagus nerve: The longest nerve in the autonomic nervous system, originating in the brainstem and branching out to various organs, acting as the primary route for the parasympathetic system's signals of relaxation and recovery; the body's built-in, rest-and-digest pathway.

Valerian: A herb known for its deep, settling properties, resonating with the Root chakra (use with care).

Vata: One of the three *doshas* in Ayurveda, representing the elements of Air and Space, associated with movement, creativity and change.

Vikriti: In Ayurvedic philosophy, a state of imbalance or disease.

Vishuddha: The Sanskrit name for the Throat chakra, meaning 'especially pure'.

Volatile aroma compounds: The aromatic molecules in essential oils which travel to the olfactory system when inhaled.

Volatile organic compounds: Chemical compounds found in essential oils which contribute to their therapeutic properties.

Wellness: The positive pursuit of harmonious balance across the multiple dimensions of life, including physical, mental, emotional, social and spiritual well-being.

Witch Craze: A horrific historical era of slaughter between the 14th and 18th centuries across Europe, where an estimated 80,000 women, including healers, herbalists, and midwives, were put to death.

Wound healing: A therapeutic effect of essential oils, particularly noted by Jean Valmet during the Second World War.

Yin and Yang: In Traditional Chinese Medicine: opposing, yet complementary, forces whose balance is essential for health and harmony.

Ylang ylang: An aromatic, floral essential oil that resonates with the Sacral chakra, supporting emotional flow, sensory relaxation and creativity.

Benham, J. *The Creamy Craft of Cosmetic Making with Essential Oils and Their Friends.* Aroma Shoppe. ISBN: 9781907571190. Published: 2011.

Blamey, Marjorie & Christopher Grey-Wilson. *Wild Flowers of the Mediterranean.* Collins. ISBN: 9780002192880. Published: 1979.

Bremness, Lesley. *World of Herbs.* Ebury Press. ISBN: 9780852239216. Published: 1990.

Brooke, Elisabeth. *A Woman's Book of Herbs.* Aeon Books Ltd. ISBN: 9781911597223. Published: 2018.

Carr-Gomm, Philip & Stephanie Carr-Gomm. *The Druid Plant Oracle.* St. Martin's Press. ISBN: 9780312369774. Published: 2008.

Chown, Vicky & Kim Walker. *The Handmade Apothecary: Healing Herbal Remedies.* Sterling Ethos. ISBN: 9781454930662. Published: 2018.

Cunningham, Scott. *Cunningham's Encyclopedia of Magical Herbs.* Llewellyn Publications. ISBN: 9780875421223. Published: 1985.

Culpeper, Nicholas. *Culpeper's Complete Herbal.* Foulsham. ISBN: 9780572002039. Published: 1995.

Herbalists Without Borders Bristol. *The Herbal Year Book.* Active Distribution. ISBN: 9781914567179. Published: 2022.

Jones, Alick & Sarah. *The Fascination of Weeds.* ISBN: 978 184 963 936 1. Austen Macauley Publishers Ltd. Published: 2015.

Kirkby, Mandy. *The Language of Flowers: A Miscellany.* Macmillan. ISBN: 9780230759633. Published: 2011.

Lawless, Julia. *The Encyclopedia of Essential Oils.* HarperCollins Publishers. ISBN: 9780007145188. Published: 2014.

Lyth, Geoff & Sue Charles. *Aromatherapy Lexicon.* Amberwood Publishing. ISBN: 9781899308156. Published: 1997.

McVicar, Jekka. *Jekka's Complete Herb Book.* Hachette UK. ISBN: 9781856267809. Published: 2009.

Papiomytoglou, Vangelis & Nikos Nikitidis. *Green Plants & Herbs of Greece.* Mediterraneo Editions. ISBN: 9789606848438. Published: 2011.

Pole, Sebastian. *Cleanse, Nurture, Restore with Herbal Tea.* White Lion Publishing. ISBN: 9780711238299. Published: 2017.

Price, Shirley. *Practical Aromatherapy.* Thorsons Publishers. ISBN: 9780722528501. Published: 1994.

Royal Botanic Gardens Kew. *The Gardener's Companion to Medicinal Plants.* Quarto Publishing PLC. ISBN: 9780711238107. Published: 2017.

Sauer, Walter. *How to Identify Flowering Plant Families.* Timber Press. ISBN: 9780917304217. Published: 1982.

Shealy, C. Norman. *The Illustrated Encyclopedia of Healing Remedies.* HarperCollins Publishers LTD. ISBN: 9780007749638. Published: 2002.

Simpson, Liz. *The Book of Chakra Healing.* Octopus Publishing Group. ISBN: 9780753731055. Published: 2016.

Toll, Maia. *The Illustrated Herbiary: Guidance and Rituals from 36 Bewitching Botanicals.* Storey Publishing. ISBN: 9781612129686. Published: 2018.

Tsouctidi, Catherine. *Greek Herbs: From Ancient Times to Today.* Privately Published. ISBN: 9786180016027. Published: 2019.

Warner, Monica. *Flowers of Jamaica.* Macmillan Caribbean. ISBN: 9780333975237. Published: 2004.

Warner, Monica. *Herbal Plants of Jamaica.* Macmillan Caribbean. ISBN: 9781405065665. Published: 2007.

Worwood, Valerie Ann. *The Fragrant Pharmacy: A Home and Health Care Guide to Aromatherapy and Essential Oils.* Bantam. ISBN: 9780553403978. Published: 1991.

van Wyk, Ben-Erik & Michael Wink. *Medicinal Plants of the World.* CABI. ISBN: 9781786393258. Published: 2017.

Wong, James. *Grow Your Own Drugs.* BBC Books. ISBN: 9780007845484. Published: 2009.

Acknowledgements

I would particularly like to thank the following beautiful souls who have helped me walk the journey of this book:

My publisher, Shirley McLellan, with thanks and gratitude for her support, patience and sheer hard graft in making such a good job of it.

Jo Thomas, my lifelong friend who illustrated the beautiful botanicals, and helped shape my thinking and selection process through our creative Devon retreats.

Another lifelong friend, Lucy Jacobs, who always listens and never judges, and has an incredible skill of asking the right questions and helping me to talk through the answers.

My tiny dancer and extraordinary artist, Melody Alexander, for her affirmation and constant joyful kindness.

My wonderful children, Kia and Joe, for their constant inspiration and love.

About the Illustrator

The illustrations in this book were created by UK artist Jo Thomas. She and Tamara grew up together in Reading and have known each other for nearly 50 years.

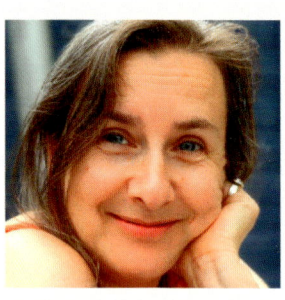

Jo also works balancing energies in homes and on land as a house healer and dowser, having had a long interest in the subtle energies of place.

'I was delighted when Tamara asked if I could be involved in her project and have the opportunity to spend time with plants and reflect on the healing they bring us.

The images are drawn from plants I've spent time with. The plants found their way to me through friends, family, local places I love as well as the creative retreats Tamara and I enjoyed at my home in Devon as the book took shape.

I've been inspired by the stories Tamara has gathered, the personal and mythic. I was struck by how often the feminine becomes embodied within the plant and that in the bloom, the healing is found.'

Jo can be found at www.presencingplace.net